YOUR APPETITE

'I really loved Phase 1. I contin[...]
Phase 1 and was rewarded with [...]
great deal of effor[...]

'I had eaten more in five days than I used to eat in a month, so I got on the scales at the end of the first week with scepticism. Man, was I in for a shock . . . A week on the Special K diet lost me 1lb, a week on Phase 1 lost me 6lb. It was a miracle, and I've not looked back since.' *Lizzi*

'I lost an amazing 9lb in five days, followed by another 5lb in the following week and seeing a stone disappear so quickly was a fabulous boost.' *Cazbah*

'What a revelation. I started this diet to lose weight, within two weeks I was continuing on it for my health. Thank you Zoë.' *Tracie*

'The best sort of diet is one that never lets you get hungry and this is the best diet for that.' *Sue15cat*

'I did Phase 1 for five days. The cravings magically went, which is fantastic. I felt that I was now in control of what I was eating rather than my cravings controlling me. This has lasted in Phase 2.' *Julie*

'For me it is all about health. I have never felt better.' *Carol*

'What an amazing way of eating – no counting, just eating real food. No more feelings of desperation and guilt from bingeing.'
Gettingslimmer

'I just dived in to Phase 1! I was stunned to have lost 8lb with no real trauma and eating all sorts of foods that I had avoided for years – amazing! Phase 2 is cool and I can eat like this forever. I've never felt better and never been so relaxed about food – Zoë, you're a marvel!' *Woofighter*

'When I weighed on the morning after day five, I had lost 10lb! I emerged into my next five day phase feeling so in control of my eating and better than I have done in years. I know that this is my eating habit for the rest of my life. I have lost all my cravings and I am particularly loving the side effects of that – losing weight and feeling 10 years younger!' *Jans*

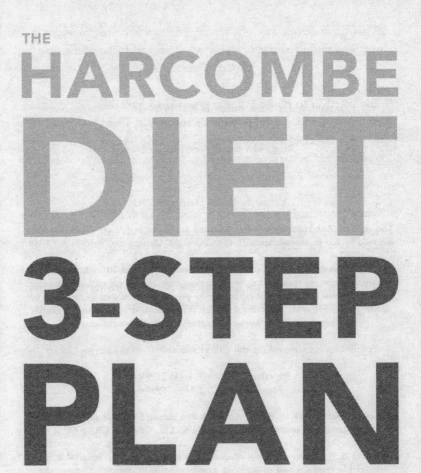

THE HARCOMBE DIET 3-STEP PLAN

Zoë Harcombe

HODDER

First published in Great Britain in 2013 by Hodder & Stoughton
An Hachette UK company

First published in paperback in 2014

1

A CIP catalogue record for this title is available from the British Library

Paperback ISBN 978 1 444 76989 0
Ebook ISBN 978 1 444 76990 6

Typeset in Sabon MT by Palimpsest Book Production Ltd, Falkirk, Stirlingshire
Printed and bound by CPI Group (UK) Ltd, Croydon CR0 4YY

Hodder & Stoughton policy is to use papers that are natural, renewable and
recyclable products and made from wood grown in sustainable forests. The
logging and manufacturing processes are expected to conform to the
environmental regulations of the country of origin.

Hodder & Stoughton Ltd
338 Euston Road
London NW1 3BH

www.hodder.co.uk

THANK YOU . . .

Thank you to the growing number of followers of The Harcombe Diet® for trusting nature to feed you better than food manufacturers. Thank you for your emails, letters, testimonials and questions. Thank you for encouraging others to start eating food – we shouldn't need to call it real food. Thank you especially for your tips, experiences and heart-warming success stories, which you have so generously shared in this book.

To find out more . . .

www.zoeharcombe.com
www.theharcombediet.com
www.theharcombedietclub.com
www.theobesityepidemic.org

CONTENTS

HOW THE HARCOMBE DIET
CAME ABOUT

My childhood dream was to go to Cambridge University. I went to the kind of school where no pupil went to Cambridge, not even on the bus! Yet I achieved my goal, winning a scholarship to read economics at Corpus Christi College. After dreaming for so long of studying at the most beautiful institution in the world, you would imagine that my time at Cambridge was everything I had hoped it would be and more. This was sadly not the case.

What should have been the time of my life was marred by the terrible relationship that I had with food. It didn't help that the Timotei shampoo model was in my year! Along with many other gorgeous 'Sloane Rangers', who were all the rage at the time. Varying between 10 and 30lb (5–14kg) heavier than the natural weight I am now, I felt fat and unattractive.

Far worse than this, I felt absolutely and completely out of control around food. I wanted to be slim more than anything else in the world. I started each day resolutely determined that I would stick to whatever I had told myself I would eat that day and yet I hardly ever managed to stick to my plan.

My idea of a 'good' day, by the way, was four large Red Delicious apples and a box (100g) of fruit gums. Fat-free and approximately 700 calories. No wonder I couldn't stick to that. My body must have been crying out for the 13 vitamins and approximately 16 minerals that it needs to keep me alive, hardly any of which are present in apples, let alone those sweets. A 'bad' day could easily involve a few cream cakes/croissants from the famous Fitzbillies cake shop (right next to Corpus Christi College for some reason);

endless sweets and chocolate munched throughout the day; meals in the college dining hall (which I tried to avoid on 'good' days) and a few bags of crisps in the evening.

I felt hopeless, helpless, out of control, scared and completely baffled. I was bright and determined. I could achieve seemingly anything I set out to achieve – Cambridge admission – but I could not control my eating. Out of this feeling of despair came a drive to understand what was going on.

My passion at school had always been maths and I found myself choosing the maths options throughout the economics course. And to me, this became the ultimate problem to solve – why did I overeat when all I wanted was to be slim?

The discovery of The Harcombe Diet became a long journey throughout my twenties. It was a journey to answer the question that became the title of my first book: *Why do you overeat? When all you want is to be slim.*

The first discovery was made while at Cambridge. I went to the doctor on the college campus, not really expecting any practical help. Thankfully, I was wrong. I took along a list of bizarre symptoms: gaining or losing pounds literally overnight; bloating; food cravings; mood swings; feeling foggy, like I was sleepwalking, all the time and more. I met the first doctor who did not dismiss me as a neurotic female. He referred me to the UK centre of excellence for Food Intolerance – at Addenbrooke's Hospital in Cambridge, as luck would have it.

FOOD INTOLERANCE – This means, quite simply, not being able to tolerate a particular food. Food Intolerance develops when you have too much of a food, too often, and your body just gets to the point where it can't cope with that food any longer. Food Intolerance can make a person feel really unwell.

> The key symptoms of Food Intolerance include bloating; irritable bowel syndrome; dramatic fluctuations in weight from one day to the next; cravings for very specific foods; eating some foods to the exclusion of others; muscle aches; thirst; coated tongue; flushed cheeks and more.

I had the added good fortune of being seen by one of the UK's leading Food Intolerance experts personally, Dr Jonathan Brostoff, and he put me on an elimination diet to take me off all likely suspect foods. The basic diet included meat, fish, eggs, vegetables, fruit, brown rice and not much else. The benefit for me was twofold. First, I added into my diet nutrient-dense foods that I had simply not been eating with my low fat/low calorie binge/starve pattern. Second, I stopped all sugar, white flour and processed food, in which I so often indulged on 'bad' days.

The transformation was instant and incredible. I dropped approximately 10lb (5kg) in a fortnight. The bloating disappeared, as did the foggy feeling, energy highs and lows and all the other nasty ailments. I felt like a new person. At this moment, I thought that I had solved the puzzle. I knew that I overate because I had been intolerant to some foods and I learned that we crave the foods to which we are intolerant. This is because of stage three of the four stages of addiction: we feel bad when we don't have the substance, so this drives us to make sure that we do consume it.

THE FOUR STAGES OF ADDICTION
1) We crave a particular substance
2) We want more and more of that substance
3) We get to the point where we feel bad when we don't have that particular substance
4) We suffer consequences as a result of the substance – weight gain being the most common consequence of food addiction

I really thought that was it – problem solved. The million dollar question has been answered. But it was nowhere near as easy as that.

I did quite well sticking to a basic foods diet for a couple of years, but I found myself eating more and more fruit. I could eat fruit to the exception of almost anything else. While working in London, after graduation, there was a fruit stall at Charing Cross Station, a couple of minutes' walk from my office on the Strand, and I would shop there at least once a day. I would return to the office with pounds of dates, cherries, apples and grapes and consume them all at my desk. I was still counting calories at this stage, so I figured that a pound of cherries, apples and grapes accounted for approximately 250, 225 and 300 calories respectively – fewer than 800. I could thus graze on fruit all day long and still be well under that magic 1000 calorie a day diet.

I conveniently forgot the pounds of dates that I used to buy as well – worse – the medjool variety. These add up to 1250 calories per pound, but I refused to believe this. Everyone knows that fruit is super healthy and fat-free, so the calorie tables must be wrong. There goes the mind-set of an addict and I was an addict. Medjool dates were my ultimate crave food. I would drive out of my way on the way home, often by miles, to get my fix. I remember the joy of the advent of 24-hour shopping, turning up at a supermarket early on a Monday morning to get my 'drugs' before work, only to find that the shops didn't open until 8am on Monday. The panic that set in was palpable.

This is when the second condition started to manifest itself. As my brother had developed type 1 diabetes as a teenager, I had regularly been tested for diabetes by family doctors and I was very familiar with the mood and energy swings that accompany blood glucose level instability. Diabetes is also known as *hyper*glycaemia – defined as high blood glucose. I was not familiar with the term *hypo*glycaemia – low blood glucose. I was, however, experiencing it on a daily basis.

The sugar that I was consuming in my fruit consumption was astronomical. Along with it went massive bloating – I would be sitting at my desk with my stomach expanding by the hour. By the end of the day I was so uncomfortable that I would have happily changed into jogging bottoms, had I not been required to be a snappy city worker in suits, stockings and heels.

Cravings for sugar didn't stop there. Despite all the things that I had learned from Dr Brostoff, sweets generally had crept back into my diet – fruit gums, chewy humbugs (they last a long time), chocolate – any confectionery was proving too tempting to resist. It took a period of working in the USA to discover why . . .

Working abroad in one's twenties sounds glamorous, but it can be very lonely. My twenties followed the Wall Street/Gordon Gekko era where 'lunch was for wimps' and my early work experience was epitomised by submissions of time sheets totalling junior doctor kinds of hours. My record time sheet submitted for one week was 105 hours – that's seven 15-hour days.

One rare evening off, I was wandering around a mall and popped into a book shop, not least because it had a cappuccino bar and I fancied a milky coffee and a bran muffin (bran – it must be healthy). As I browsed the book shop, a title jumped out at me: *New Low Blood Sugar and You* by Carlton Fredericks. The back cover had been written for me: 'anxiety, irritability, exhaustion, fainting spells, headaches, indigestion, indecisiveness, forgetfulness . . .' I had actually passed out on a couple of occasions, which had been very scary. I settled down to read the book and was just blown away. The energy and mood highs and lows, the constant cravings for sugary foods, the constant jitteriness (I hadn't thought of it as anxiety) I suffered being so hyper on sugar all the time – all suddenly had an explanation.

HYPOGLYCAEMIA – Literally a Greek translation from *hypo*, meaning 'under', *glykis*, meaning 'sweet' and *emia*, meaning 'in the blood'. The three bits all put together mean low blood 'sugar' (glucose). Hypoglycaemia describes the state the body is in if your blood glucose levels are too low. When your blood glucose levels are too low, this is potentially life threatening and your body will try to get you to eat.

Hypoglycaemia can develop when we consume too much glucose, too often, and place excessive demands on our body to release the right amount of insulin every time to return our blood glucose level to normal. If we release too much or too little insulin, blood glucose levels remain outside the normal range. This delicate mechanism within the body was not designed to cope with the modern diet of cereal/toast for breakfast, sandwiches/crisps for lunch, pasta/potatoes for dinner and cakes, biscuits, confectionery and crisps in between. All carbohydrates break down into sugars and our current diet is a recipe for Hypoglycaemia.

The key symptoms of Hypoglycaemia include energy and mood swings; irritability; inability to concentrate; indecisiveness; feeling shaky or faint; waking in the early hours and not being able to get back to sleep; cravings for sugar and caffeine; weight gain; 'get up and go' has got up and gone.

For the next couple of years, I tried desperately to overcome sugar cravings, but I just couldn't seem to go more than a couple of days without fruit – a couple of hours some days. I felt like I had the solution, but just couldn't put it into practice.

The final piece in the jigsaw proved to be another book, in another book store – this time back in London. I was browsing the books in Holland & Barrett, a health store, and Leon

Chaitow's *Candida Albicans: Could Yeast Be Your Problem?* called out to me. The words were on the front cover this time: 'anxiety, irritability, bloatedness, heartburn, tiredness, allergies, cystitis, menstrual problems . . .' An incredible overlap with the book on Hypoglycaemia, and with a couple more symptoms on top. Yes – this described me.

CANDIDA – A yeast, which lives in all of us, and is normally kept under control by our immune system and other bacteria in our body. It usually lives in the digestive system. Candida has no useful purpose. If it stays in balance, it causes no harm. If it multiplies out of control, it can create havoc with every aspect of our health.

The key symptoms of Candida include bloating; irritable bowel syndrome; feeling 'spaced out'; water retention; cravings for sugary/yeasty/vinegary foods; athlete's foot; thrush; dandruff; fatigue; and these symptoms worsen on damp/rainy days.

The overlap intrigued me, so I bought the Chaitow book and a couple of others that I found on the subject of Candida. I went home and got out the books on Food Intolerance, Hypoglycaemia and Candida – quite a collection by this time – and I set to work.

The floor in my small London flat was soon covered in books, wedged open at different pages, and pieces of paper with my scribbles. I looked at causes and symptoms of, and solutions for, the three conditions and could not quite believe the overlap.

Quite mathematically, I went through what was allowed on the perfect diet to overcome each condition. Many had different diet stages, so I wanted to discover the shortest period of time in which a difference could be made. This turned out to be driven by Food Intolerance. It takes three to four days for a digested substance to pass through our bodies and so we can be comfortably free from a potential Food Intolerance substance after five days.

Hypoglycaemia can be massively helped in as little as one day – avoid all sugars and reduce carbohydrate intake dramatically for even one day and blood glucose levels will stabilise remarkably quickly. Candida proved to be the condition that would take much longer to overcome – weeks, or even months in some extreme cases.

I simply worked out the lowest common denominator for all bits of advice – the base diet that each condition would allow – and this became the perfect diet to overcome the three conditions that cause insatiable food cravings. Thus The Harcombe Diet was born.

The final question in the puzzle to ask and answer was 'why did I get these three conditions?' Why did I become a condition driven food addict?

The final piece in the jigsaw was a show stopper. I got these three conditions because I had been dieting – calorie counting to be precise. I started trying to lose weight at the age of 15 and became an obsessive calorie counter within weeks of starting a calorie controlled diet. Nothing mattered to me, except trying to eat less (and trying to do more as often as possible without physically collapsing). I did lose weight at first, but not the promised 2lb (1kg) a week, week in, week out. It wasn't long before weight loss stopped and I found that I had to eat less and less to try to induce any further weight loss. I was a 16 year old – playing hockey, tennis, rounders and athletics for the school, working as a lifeguard, training for further lifesaving qualifications, playing the clarinet and piano to Grade 8 level and taking O-Levels – on no more than 1000 calories a day. I would take four small apples and two slices of dry bread to school for lunch. Before long, I'd realised that I could save 150 calories a day if I threw the bread to the birds at lunch time.

Even without being able to avoid a family dinner in the evening, I could often get away with 600–800 calories a day. I got to the point that I would gain weight eating any more than this.

What I didn't know at the time was that I was setting myself up for the three conditions beautifully:

1 Candida

The weakened immune system alone, from months of eating too little, had caused Candida. My chosen diet foods of fruit, crispbreads, vinegar – not oil – on salads, fat free sweets, etc, had fuelled Candida further.

2 Food Intolerance

Calorie counters need to get 'the biggest bang for the buck' – the most food for the fewest calories – otherwise the sense of deprivation is intolerable. I ate the same things every day – the same calorie counted cereal, the same bread, the same coleslaw and low calorie salad dressing, even the same type of apple (Granny Smith). Food Intolerance is, by definition, eating too much of the same thing and too often – that's how calorie counters get Food Intolerance.

3 Hypoglycaemia

Because, as a calorie counter, I had shunned fat (why have fat with approximately nine calories per gram when you can have carbs with approximately four calories per gram?) I had inevitably embraced carbs instead. Eating carbs impacts blood glucose levels and makes the calorie counter more likely to be lurching from one sugar high to the next or one sugar low to the next. Worse, as a calorie counter, I was continuously grazing. To make the hunger more manageable, I tried to eat all the time – making a fruit gum last as long as possible, cutting an apple into tiny pieces and making it seem like a meal. Calorie counters are the ultimate grazers and they are, therefore, messing up blood glucose levels the whole time.

The calorie counter is virtually guaranteed to develop the three conditions that cause insatiable cravings. It is no coincidence that calorie deficit dieters cannot maintain their weight loss – the cravings are so overwhelming, try as the dieter might, they cannot resist the urge to eat. The former calorie counter is absolutely determined to stay slim, but they are now also a food addict, with virtually no chance of resisting the many drivers to eat.

You may well be familiar with this situation – you lost weight, were determined to keep it off, and then biscuits, crisps and/or chocolate were 'talking to you' and you just couldn't silence them. You gave in – just today, only today – determined that you would be back on track tomorrow. However, giving in to the biscuits, crisps and/or chocolate nicely fed Candida, nicely embedded Food Intolerance and nicely continued your Hypoglycaemia. You woke up the next day just as likely to crave and binge on processed carbohydrates as the day before. And the day after. And so on.

It is not your fault that you lost some weight, but couldn't keep it off. Now you know – counting calories turned you into a food addict. On The Harcombe Diet you won't eat less and you won't develop the three conditions. On the contrary, you are doing the perfect diet to overcome the three conditions and to make sure that you end food addiction forever. This is why you are only ever going to start one last diet: The Harcombe Diet.

THE HEADLINES

Having read every diet book under the sun, I know that all you want right now are the headlines. How much will I lose? What can I eat? Is this workable for me? So here goes:

★ The strictest phase of the diet, Phase 1, is only five days long (although we will encourage those of you with more to lose to stay on this for longer for the best results). A typical day would be bacon and eggs for breakfast, Salade Niçoise for lunch and curry and brown rice for dinner.

★ The main weight loss part of the diet, Phase 2, allows steak, cheese, whole grains, fruit. It's not low calorie, it's not low fat and it's not low carb.

★ Lifelong weight maintenance, Phase 3, will teach you how to enjoy chocolate, wine, creamy desserts, crisps and ice cream – The Harcombe Diet way.

★ You can do this as a vegetarian – I was a vegetarian for approximately 20 years, including the time I designed and followed the diet to reach and maintain my own natural weight.

★ You don't need to exercise to lose weight. In fact, sometimes exercise can be *unhelpful* for weight loss – we'll explain how. Weight loss is about *what* you put in your mouth – not even how much you put in your mouth – and it's *not* about what you do.

★ The record weight loss in the first five days is 17lb (8kg). People with a lot to lose typically lose 7–10lb (3–5kg). Even those with less to lose often lose 3–5lb (1–2kg) in Phase 1.

★ You'll start this diet to lose weight. You'll stay on it because you're about to feel healthier than you can ever remember.

GETTING READY FOR THE LAST DIET YOU'LL EVER NEED

It is estimated that 15 million people in the UK alone are on a diet at any one time. Most people start a diet each Monday and rarely make it past Wednesday. It is further estimated that eight out of ten women and seven out of ten men start a diet on New Year's Day.

As so many people have discovered, The Harcombe Diet really is the last diet that you will ever need to start. It will be a lifestyle change that you adopt from this point onwards – something that works, which you can stick to and enjoy and the food that you indulge in will leave you in great shape and health. However, I appreciate that you're probably carrying a bit of baggage, having tried every other diet before this one. So here are the three things that you need to do to ensure that this really is the last diet you ever start:

1 Get your mind ready

Understandably, if you've switched from one calorie restricted diet to another, and none have ever worked, you would quite rightly expect the next low calorie diet not to work. And it won't. Know that whatever you try next must allow you to eat enough to feel great and to make sure that nothing slows down your metabolism ever again.

If you have tried low carbohydrate diets and found them too restrictive and miserable to stick to, you have at least picked up an appreciation for the power of carbohydrate management. This has been a great lesson to learn, but you now know that whatever you try next must allow you to eat more than skinless chicken breasts for days on end.

Your mind needs to have learned something from all the 'failures' in the past. We usually learn far more from things that haven't worked than from things that have worked, so be glad for all your experiences to date and make sure that none of the pain that you went through is wasted.

When you realise that low calorie diets don't work and low carbohydrate diets can be too tough to stick to, you're ready to try something completely different. The Harcombe Diet is so different that you have every reason to believe that it will work for you. Start this diet with the commitment that this time you plan to work *with* your body and have it work back with you. No more starvation, no more calorie counted processed food, no more dietary fat phobia, just real food, three times a day and plenty of nourishment.

2 Get your body ready

So many people have a last binge before starting a diet – 'I'll lose it all tomorrow' is the thinking. This is possibly the worst thing that you can do. You want to get your body ready to work with you, not fighting you because you've just stuffed it full of things that it doesn't recognise. The day before a diet you should actually be trying to get all the processed food that you've been eating out of your system and then you're ready to start eating well with stable blood glucose levels, not a binge hangover.

Some people read the book and start that day. Some people even come across The Harcombe Diet online, download a free 10-day plan and start that minute without knowing anything about the three conditions or why the diet works. Such people start the diet without having had a last binge and they can do really well. However, if you're a more 'plan ahead' type of person, and you are diligently reading this book in preparation for arranging a start date, please start taking on board the principles as soon as you read about them. Start ditching processed food as soon as you know the difference between fake and real food. Start feeling bad about the lengths that food manufacturers will go to, to make you desire their substances. Start vowing to be nice to yourself from now on, and being nice means nourishing yourself with great food. Bingeing on confectionery is *not* being nice to yourself and it needs to stop.

Some of the best tips from our Harcombe followers are about cutting back on caffeine even before starting Phase 1. Many suffered caffeine withdrawal more than anything else during Phase 1 and their experiences can really help you.

So, please *don't* have that last binge. Junk food isn't going away. It will be there every day for the rest of your life. It's not as though if you don't have it today, you can never have it again. You can have junk any time you like. Just give it five days and your desire for 'forbidden' foods is going to have subsided massively. The goal of The Harcombe Diet is to get you to the point that processed food holds no interest for you as quickly as we possibly can. Incredible as it may seem now, the junk that you're craving today will hold no power over you once you get these three conditions under control.

3 Get your kitchen ready

The right food has to be in your home and the wrong food has to be out of your home – it's as simple as that. If you are going to follow The Harcombe Diet menu plans, have a shopping list ready and have everything you need until your next shop. If you only need to do a five day Phase 1, then you can shop for five days if you are able to stock up on day four. If you shop once a week habitually, then make sure you stock up for a full week – don't risk getting caught out.

If you are happy looking at the list of allowed foods and are planning to do your own flexi plan to suit your lifestyle and preferences, again, have the meals planned and groceries in your home ready.

Your cupboards need tinned fish, tinned tomatoes, olive oil, brown rice, quinoa, oats, oat biscuits and a good selection of herbs and spices. Eggs are best kept somewhere cool, but not in the fridge. The fridge needs vegetables, salads, natural live yoghurt, butter, milk and cheese, depending on which Phase you are in. Meat and fish for the next couple of days should be in the omnivore's fridge and options are best kept in the freezer for the longer term. Freezers are also great for stocking up on berries in season and having them out of season.

Whatever you are planning to bring into the home, it is equally important to get the wrong food out of sight. Be ruthless. If you live alone then empty the freezer, cupboards and fridge of any and all temptations. Don't hang on to biscuits 'in case I have a visitor'. The visitor doesn't need them either. Throw things away, making sure that they cannot be retrieved later from the dustbin. Yes – we've all been there!

If you live with others, you need to enlist their support. Ideally, flatmates or family members can join you. Even if they don't need to lose weight, most people need to gain health. If you are the household cook, then you determine the meals. If someone else wants a ready meal, let them stick it in the microwave. Let them know that you will be roasting meat, stir-frying vegetables, knocking up some fabulous curries and tasty dishes, but you won't be joining them in having a takeaway or making sandwiches.

If other people want crisps, biscuits, ice cream and so on in the home and won't support you in getting rid of this just to help you through the early stages of the diet, then you need to forgive them for their addiction. You will need to be extra strong to ignore the junk within reach and to have your healthy meals instead. This is where the 'get your mind ready' is so important. At the point you start the diet you need to be absolutely resolute that this is it. This is the last one. This is the one that is going to work. With every day that passes, the cravings will subside and this strength will be tested less and less as time goes by.

PHASE 1

THE KICK START FOR RAPID WEIGHT LOSS

EVERYTHING YOU NEED TO KNOW ABOUT PHASE 1

Phase 1 is just five days long. As we covered in 'How The Harcombe Diet came about', the length of Phase 1 is determined by the condition Food Intolerance. Phase 1 will always be five days long, by design, for this reason.

However, experience has shown that some people should stay on Phase 1 for longer than five days to optimise their weight loss success. We are, therefore, introducing a new concept in this book to make sure that The Harcombe Diet works better than ever for you.

There are two particular groups of people that should stay on Phase 1 for longer than five days and you may be in either or both groups:

1 Those with more weight to lose

2 Those with moderate or severe Candida, as this condition takes more than a few days to get under control

For (1) you are going to fall into one of three broad guideline weight loss groups: Do you have less than 20lb (9kg) to lose? Are you in the 20–50lb (9–23kg) range? Do you have more than 50lb (23kg) to lose? Most people will know intuitively which of these three groups they fall into. Here is how to check:

• The Body Mass Index, BMI, is not perfect, but it is a useful guide to see how close to our natural weight we might be. (Our natural weight is the weight that we find we can maintain quite easily – we'll cover this in more detail throughout the book). Put 'BMI calculator' into an internet search engine and you will find a tool that will calculate your current BMI for you.

- Enter your height – the best BMI calculators will let you do this in metric (metres and centimetres) or imperial (feet and inches), as suits you. Enter your weight; again, ideally you will be given an option of entering your details in metric (kilograms) or imperial (pounds).
- The official guidelines are that a BMI below 18.5 is underweight, a BMI of 18.5–24.9 is normal weight, a BMI of 25–29.9 is overweight, a BMI of 30 or above is obese.
- Estimate which weight loss group you are in: less than 20lb (9kg) to lose; 20–50lb (9–23kg) to lose or more than 50lb (23kg) to lose. Deduct the weight that you think you have to lose from your current weight and then re-enter this as your weight in the BMI calculator. This will tell you what your BMI would be if you reached this weight. If your 'target' weight results in a BMI of 20 or below, this is *unlikely* to be your natural weight, so you will likely have less to lose than you estimated. If your 'target' weight gives a BMI of approximately 21–27, this may well be your natural weight range. We will discuss BMI and natural weight more later on in the book (taller people tend to have natural weights that give slightly higher BMI readings, while many men, especially former athletes, end up in the 'overweight' BMI category and yet look fit, slim and optimally healthy).

As an example, let's say you are 5ft 4in (163cm) and 12 stone (76kg); this means that you will enter 64in (163cm) and 168lb (76kg) into the BMI calculator. This will tell you that you have a BMI of 28.8 – in the overweight category. If you lost 20lb (9kg) and entered 64in (163cm) for height and 148lb (67kg) for weight) you would have a BMI of 25.4 – just slightly in the overweight category. So you are likely to be in the 20–50lb (9–23kg) to lose category. Another 5ft 4in (163cm) woman weighing 10 stone (63kg) would have a BMI of 24. This woman would be in the less than 20lb (9kg) to lose category and may in fact be quite close to her natural weight already.

The second thing to determine is how mild, moderate or severe your Candida overgrowth is, and the following questionnaire/table will help you.

SYMPTOMS OF THE THREE CONDITIONS

When I discovered the three conditions that cause insatiable food cravings, I was struck by the similarity of symptoms related to Candida, Food Intolerance and Hypoglycaemia. I have read extensively on all three conditions, covering the original works on each, and the overlapping symptoms are numerous.

In the following table, symptoms are grouped into those common to gastric/stomach problems, headaches and physical symptoms related to the head, psychological and mood complaints and so on. Every symptom listed in the table is a symptom of Candida. The problems related to Candida are the most varied and extensive of all three conditions.

The table thus has a column for symptoms unique to Candida, that is, symptoms *not* related to Food Intolerance and/or Hypoglycaemia. There is then a column for where symptoms of Food Intolerance overlap with Candida and a column for where symptoms of Hypoglycaemia overlap with Candida.

This table is going to be your key monitoring tool as you progress with The Harcombe Diet. You may like to photocopy the table a few times so that you can date each copy as you track changes.

Before you start Phase 1, go through the table and please tick every symptom that you currently experience. Make a note of whether you would describe the symptom as mild, moderate or severe, using the following descriptions:*

MILD = I rarely experience this symptom – maybe every now and again, but not even once a week; and/or when I do experience this symptom, it doesn't really trouble me.

MODERATE = I quite often experience this symptom – at least a couple of times a week; and/or when I do experience this symptom, it troubles me to the point of discomfort.

SEVERE = I often experience this symptom – daily or more frequently; and/or when I do experience this symptom, it is really quite disabling.

Before you start Phase 1, if you tick any of the symptoms that are common to more than one condition, you won't be able to tell which condition is causing the problem. If you have bloating, irritable bowel syndrome and other stomach problems, for example, you won't know if you are suffering from Candida or Food Intolerance, or both. If you are suffering from symptoms in the blood glucose category and/or symptoms in the mind and mood section, you won't know which of the three conditions has caused this.

The biggest clue as to your level of Candida overgrowth before starting Phase 1 is going to come from the symptoms unique to Candida. Thrush (yeast infections), athlete's foot, dandruff, feeling noticeably worse on damp days – these are going to be your key indicators of Candida overgrowth. Rate any symptoms unique to Candida as mild, moderate or severe and you will have a useful starting assessment for this condition.

---

* Please use the *frequency* with which you experience the symptom and the *severity* of the symptom as a guide.

After five days of Phase 1, you will be able to redo this questionnaire to get a clear indication of the extent of your problem with Candida. The symptoms of Food Intolerance and Hypoglycaemia subside within a five day period. Hence, any symptoms remaining can be attributed to Candida. Rate each of them as mild, moderate and severe again, to see what you're up against.

If you have a clear trend for mostly mild, mostly moderate or mostly severe when you rate your symptoms, you've got your level of Candida established. If you've got a mixture of mild, moderate and severe, take a balanced view and level up, rather than down. For example, if you have many 'moderate' and some 'mild' and some 'severe', assume that your Candida overgrowth is moderate overall. If you have quite a spread across mild, moderate and severe, treating your Candida as severe will be the safest option. If in doubt, assume the higher level of overgrowth. No harm will be done staying on Phase 1 longer and it will be better to err on the side of caution and attack this nasty parasite.

Redo the questionnaire regularly to see how you are doing in getting Candida back under control. Any time you see the symptoms coming back, rather than going away, you should return to Phase 1 as the perfect diet to overcome all three conditions.

The conditions questionnaire

Symptoms (NB all symptoms listed are signs of Candida)	Unique to Candida	Food Intolerance	Hypoglycaemia
Stomach Constipation		x	

THE HARCOMBE DIET 3-STEP PLAN

Symptoms (NB all symptoms listed are signs of Candida)	Unique to Candida	Food Intolerance	Hypoglycaemia
Diarrhoea		x	
Irritable bowel syndrome		x	
Bloating, especially after food		x	
Indigestion		x	
Gas		x	
Heartburn		x	
Head			
Headaches		x	x
Dizziness		x	x
Blurred vision			x
Flushed cheeks		x	
Feeling of 'sleepwalking'		x	x
Feeling unreal		x	x
Feeling 'spaced out'		x	x
Women			
Premenstrual tension (PMT)		x	x
Irregular periods		x	

Symptoms (NB all symptoms listed are signs of Candida)	Unique to Candida	Food Intolerance	Hypoglycaemia
Vaginal discharge or itchiness	x		
Thrush	x		
Cystitis	x		
Blood Glucose			
Hungry between meals		x	x
Irritable or moody before meals		x	x
Feeling faint/shaky when food is not eaten		x	x
Headaches late morning and late afternoon		x	x
Waking in the early hours and not being able to get back to sleep		x	x
Abnormal cravings for sweet foods, bread, alcohol or caffeine		x	x
Eating sweets makes you more hungry		x	x
Excessive appetite		x	x

THE HARCOMBE DIET 3-STEP PLAN

Symptoms (NB all symptoms listed are signs of Candida)	Unique to Candida	Food Intolerance	Hypoglycaemia
Instant sugar 'high' followed by fatigue		x	x
Chilly feeling after eating		x	x
Mind & Mood			
Anxiety		x	x
Depression		x	x
Irritability		x	x
Lethargy		x	x
Memory problems		x	x
Loss of concentration		x	x
Moodiness		x	x
Nightmares		x	x
Mental 'sluggishness'		x	x
'Get up and go' has got up and gone		x	x
Other			
Dramatic fluctuations in weight from one day to the next		x	x
Easy weight gain		x	x

EVERYTHING YOU NEED TO KNOW ABOUT PHASE 1

Symptoms (NB all symptoms listed are signs of Candida)	Unique to Candida	Food Intolerance	Hypoglycaemia
Water retention		x	
Poor circulation	x		
Hands and feet sensitive to cold	x		
Feeling of being unable to cope		x	x
Constant fatigue		x	x
Muscle aches or cramps		x	
Sighing often – 'hunger for air'		x	
Yawning easily		x	
Difficulty sleeping		x	x
Excessive thirst		x	
Coated tongue		x	
Dry skin		x	
Itchy skin/rashes		x	
Hair loss	x		
Symptoms worse after consuming yeasty or sugary foods		x	

Symptoms (NB all symptoms listed are signs of Candida)	Unique to Candida	Food Intolerance	Hypoglycaemia
Symptoms worse on damp, humid or rainy days	x		
Athlete's foot, dandruff or other fungal infection	x		

Once you know approximately how much weight you have to lose and how mild to severe your Candida overgrowth appears to be, please put yourself in one of the following categories to find out the recommended time for you to stay on Phase 1:

Weight to lose	Mild Candida	Moderate Candida	Severe Candida
< 20lb (9kg)	5 days	2–4 weeks	6–8 weeks
20–50lb (9–23kg)	2–4 weeks	2–4 weeks	6–8 weeks
> 50lb (23kg)	6–8 weeks	6–8 weeks	6–8 weeks

If you have less than 20lb (9kg) to lose and mild Candida, you can opt for the standard five-day Phase 1. If you have more to lose and/or more of a problem with Candida, you will really benefit from staying on Phase 1 longer. This is a recommendation rather than a rule, as there are other factors to consider. Phase 1 is more difficult for vegetarians, for example, so you may need to opt for the low end of these recommendations if you don't eat meat or fish. You may find that your lifestyle just doesn't lend itself to staying on Phase 1 of the diet longer and this may make you opt for a shorter than recommended Phase 1.

However, if you have a lot of weight to lose and/or bad Candida overgrowth, the longer you can stay on Phase 1 the better.

THE FOODS YOU CAN EAT IN PHASE 1

The foods that you can eat in Phase 1 are listed on the following pages. There are hundreds of different varieties of meat, fish and vegetables available in the natural world. All meat and fish, in their most natural form, are fine for Phase 1. All vegetables, other than potatoes and mushrooms, are fine for Phase 1. I've just listed the best known foods in what follows to give you plenty of ideas for options to try. Please see notes (1–8) after the tables for further clarification.

TABLE OF FOODS FOR PHASE 1

Vegetables

Alfalfa	Chilli (any)	Parsnip
Artichoke	Corn on the cob	Peas
Asparagus	Courgette	Pepper (any)
Aubergine	Cucumber	Pumpkin
Baby sweetcorn	Dandelion	Radish
Bamboo shoots	Endive	Rocket
Bean sprouts	Fennel	Salsify
Beetroot	Garlic	Shallot
Bok choy	Green beans	Sorrel
Broccoli	Kale	Spinach
Brussels sprouts	Leek	Spring onion
Cabbage (any)	Lettuce (any)	Squash
Carrot	Mangetout	Swede
Cauliflower	Marrow	Swiss chard
Celeriac	Mustard greens	Turnip
Celery	Okra	Water chestnuts
Chicory	Onion	Watercress

THE HARCOMBE DIET 3-STEP PLAN

Herbs & Spices

Basil	Cumin	Parsley
Bay leaves	Dill	Pepper
Caraway	Dried mixed herbs	Rosemary
Cardamom	Ginger	Saffron
Chervil	Marjoram	Sage
Chives	Mint	Salt
Cinnamon	Nutmeg	Tarragon
Cloves	Oregano	Thyme
Coriander	Paprika	Turmeric

White Fish (1)

Cod	Halibut	Sole
Coley	Monkfish	Swordfish
Haddock	Plaice	Turbot
Hake	Sea bass	Whiting

Seafood

Clams	Mussels	Scallops
Crab	Octopus	Shrimps
Crayfish	Oysters	Squid
Lobster	Prawns	Winkles

Oily Fish

Anchovies	Pilchards	Trout
Herring	Salmon	Tuna
Mackerel	Sardines	

White Meat & Birds (2)

Chicken	Guinea fowl	Rabbit
Duck	Pheasant	Turkey
Goose	Quail	

EVERYTHING YOU NEED TO KNOW ABOUT PHASE 1

Red Meat (2)

Bacon Beef Gammon	Ham Lamb Pork	Veal Venison

Offal (3)

Heart Kidneys	Liver Tongue	

Other

Brown rice, quinoa, porridge oats (4)	Natural live (bio) yoghurt (5)	Eggs (6) Tofu (7)

Fruit

Lemons/Limes	Olives	Tomato

Miscellaneous

Butter Oils (olive, sunflower,	sesame, groundnut, peanut, coconut and	other natural oils)

Drinks (8)

Any 'fruit' tea Any herbal tea	Decaf coffee Decaf tea	Water – still or sparkling

Notes from the table

1 Provided, of course, that you don't have a food allergy to any fish or seafood. Fresh, frozen or tinned fish are all fine, just no fish in breadcrumbs or fish with added ingredients.

2 Ideally get all your meat from a local butcher that you come to know and trust. Animals need to be living naturally – grazing on grass in sunlight – for meat to be optimally nutritious. If you do buy any packaged or tinned meats, please check the ingredients list carefully and avoid any with sugars (the 'oses') or other unnecessary ingredients. A preservative is the only acceptable added ingredient.

3 I appreciate that not everyone likes offal, but it is the cheapest and most nutritious food on the planet. Pregnant women in tribal communities are prioritised to be given the organ meats from animals. The whole community benefits from a healthy mum and baby, which is why this tradition has evolved.

4 The only food that is limited in quantity is the 'safe grain'. You can have up to 50g (dry weight before cooking) of brown rice, quinoa or porridge oats per day. If you are vegetarian or vegan, you can have up to 150g (dry weight before cooking) of one of these grains per day to make sure that you get enough to eat.

- The rice allowance can be used in the form of puffed brown rice cereal or brown rice pasta (literally pasta spirals made from brown rice). Both can be swapped, gram for gram dry weight, with the omnivore or vegetarian brown rice allowance. If you suffer from Hypoglycaemia, you should avoid the brown rice cereal as it will likely be too high a glycaemic food for you. For this reason, don't swap the brown rice allowance for rice cakes. They are even more 'puffed' than the cereal and could upset blood glucose levels unnecessarily. Brown rice cereal is now widely available in gluten-free sections of supermarkets. It needs to be eaten dry in Phase 1. It is the 'Marmite' of The Harcombe Diet – some people love it, some hate it. At least try it.

- Quinoa can also be swapped gram for gram with the brown rice allowance. This is a rarely eaten grain and, therefore, one of the least likely grain intolerances.

- Porridge oats are our final 'safe grain'. Avoid these if you know that you are gluten intolerant. Many people who can't tolerate wheat find that they are fine with oats and this is a really useful breakfast option, especially for people who don't eat eggs.

5 Unless you are intolerant to dairy products, you can have natural live (bio) yoghurt in Phase 1. The active cultures in live/bio yoghurt can really help with Candida overgrowth, which is why we allow this one dairy substance in Phase 1. We discuss dairy products in detail in the Phase 2 section of the book so, if you have any concern that you may be intolerant to dairy, please turn to this section and read it carefully. You will need to avoid yoghurt in Phase 1 if you think that you may be intolerant to dairy products. If you are sensitive to cow's milk, you can try a goat's or sheep's version of live yoghurt, as the health benefits of live yoghurt for Candida and the digestive tract are significant.

6 Provided that you are not intolerant to, or allergic to, eggs. Eggs should also be from animals able to graze freely on grass in the sunlight.

7 Provided that you are OK with vegetarian protein alternatives. Tofu is a soy(a) product and soy(a) is a common Food Intolerance, especially in the USA (the Americans call it soy, the Brits call it soya). Quorn is made from a type of fungus, which is not ideal for Candida, so it is best to avoid Quorn in Phase 1.

8 For drinks, you may drink as much bottled or filtered water and herbal teas as you like during Phase 1, but no alcohol, caffeine or canned drinks (even low calorie drinks) or fruit juices. You can also have any decaffeinated coffee or tea, but without milk, sugar or sweeteners. Any herbal teas are fine, even the fruit versions (like blackcurrant) – they are fruit infusions, rather than fruit itself.

The key things to avoid in Phase 1 are processed food and drinks. So no sugar, flour, sweeteners, diet drinks, packaged food, etc. You also need to avoid all grains other than the brown rice, quinoa and oats allowance. No milk or cheese and no fruit, other than the tomatoes, lemons and olives on the allowed list.

When and how much to eat
It is strongly recommended that you use Phase 1 to get into the habit of eating three meals a day. This is going to be the pattern encouraged throughout The Harcombe Diet, so the sooner you get used to this, the better. If you must snack to avoid hunger, and thus to make sure that you're not tempted by processed snack foods, then you can snack on any of the Phase 1 allowed foods: natural live yoghurt; crudités (sticks of carrot, celery, peppers, etc); hard-boiled eggs; extra meat and/or fish and so on.

To solve a weight problem, we must give our bodies the chance to burn the body fat that we are carrying. We can't do this if we are grazing like cows all day long.

With the exception of the Phase 1 'safe grains', quantities are *not* limited on The Harcombe Diet, but this doesn't mean that you eat a whole chicken at one sitting. It means that you rediscover normal eating (and it feels great when you do so).

Eat as much as you need during Phase 1, so that you don't succumb to cravings for the foods to which you have been addicted. Phase 1 should be the start of rediscovering what normal eating is. Many of us have either been starving on daft diets or bingeing on enormous quantities of junk food (or both). Phase 1 can be difficult for such 'all or nothing' types, but we need to reacquaint ourselves with how we should eat. The Phase 1 grain portion is small because none of the conditions respond well to an intake of carbohydrate higher than this. Once in Phase 2, however, your porridge serving may be nearer 100g than 50g. Meat and fish portions should *not* be the couple of ounces allowed on starvation diets. You should be enjoying 200–250g steaks covering half the plate and a mountain of vegetables covering the other half.

PHASE 1 PERSONAL EXPERIENCES

My experience with Phase 1

I'll be honest, I took a while to properly embrace Phase 1. In my defence, I was leading the way in uncharted territory. I didn't have the tens of thousands of testimonials that I have now to know that the effort would be worthwhile. In addition to this, I was an addict to end all addicts. The thought of giving up fruit for five days was just too dreadful to think about, let alone the confectionery, muffins, cheese scones (also seen as healthy), in fact anything wholemeal, which I was living on at the time. I had no desire to eat meat, fish or eggs. Why would anyone want to eat an omelette when one could have dates and a bran muffin?

I am often asked, 'What was the motivation tip that finally worked for you?' and it was this: I realised that I had to do something about my health and addiction. I knew that I couldn't continue my life lurching from one sugar high to another, bloated, continually fighting weight gain and generally feeling very unwell. I got to the point where I became aware that I had to do something about this someday, and if I was going to do something about it someday, then that someday had to be today. I realised that there was no point putting off the inevitable.

I also came to realise that these conditions don't get better. They get worse. Candida overgrowth doesn't sort itself out, it gets worse, until health can deteriorate to reach M.E. (myalgic encephalomyelitis) kinds of levels. Blood glucose levels don't stabilise on their own – the swings get wider and worse until type 2 diabetes becomes a high likelihood. Food Intolerance also doesn't correct itself. Stage three of the four stages of addiction ensures that we feel worse and worse if we don't get our fix and yet stage four ensures that we suffer more and more consequences from succumbing to the cravings. We can't win this war without the right strategy and Phase 1 is that right strategy.

So, I went home to my parents for a few days – preparing to need looking after – and what a good call that was. I have not previously shared how bad my first experience of Phase 1 was because I didn't want to put anyone off trying the diet that is going to change their life. However, I have since come to realise that no one can lose doing Phase 1. Either you sail through Phase 1 and wonder what all the fuss was about, in which case, lucky you, you caught the conditions early and you'll be a few pounds down without suffering. Or, you will think you are dying from flu and you will have the ultimate confirmation that you had one or more of the conditions by the bucket load and lucky you for starting to get these under control. It's lucky you either way.

The worse people have the conditions, the worse they tend to feel in Phase 1, but also the more weight they tend to lose.

The record weight loss is currently an incredible 17lb (8kg) and 14lb (6kg) has been lost by people on several occasions. I am personally disappointed if people don't lose 5–7lb (2–3kg). Phase 1 is quite simply your ultimate health and weight rescue remedy, which you now have with you for life.

One of the reasons that the weight loss can be so spectacular in Phase 1 is that both Candida and Food Intolerance encourage water retention. Pounds of water can be dropped quickly when the perfect diet to fight these two conditions is adopted. Some people discount water weight loss, as if only fat loss counts. The average human being is 50–60% water anyway, so you will always lose water alongside fat. If you weigh 220lb (100kg) and you should weigh 120lb (55kg), you are not going to lose 100lb

(45kg) of fat and turn into a puddle! You could be a clothes size down in just five days. Ready for that special event or just nicely back into your favourite jeans – in just five days.

Harcombe fans' experiences with Phase 1

'I found Phase 1 both easy and difficult at the same time. The food choices were easy to sustain and not worry about, but the hardest part was giving up caffeine. I was a total coffee addict and would easily have 10+ mugs a day before The Harcombe Diet. I went cold turkey and didn't think to reduce my caffeine intake gradually. Needless to say, I had severe headaches on days two and three, shakes and a general unwell feeling. By day four I was feeling so much better and by day five, felt great. I lost a whopping 15lb in those five days. I was so over the moon at such a result and couldn't wait to start Phase 2. One year on and six stone off for good!' *Josie*

'As soon as I found out bacon and eggs were a good Phase 1 breakfast I had a good feeling about this diet! I love cooked breakfasts!! For the first three days, I felt a bit lightheaded and spaced out. I also seemed to have the sweats almost like I was coming down with a cold. I still stuck to it – a typical day would be eating egg and bacon every morning, salad and tuna or salmon for lunch and griddled chicken with roasted veg for dinner. I did not feel hungry and I had no desire to snack. I also had an unhealthy relationship with wine. This craving disappeared almost immediately. Best thing about this diet is the fact it works. I lost 10lb in Phase 1. I am a mother of three with more than four stone to lose and the cliché goes, "If I can do it, anyone can," but I really mean that!!' *Kayla*

'I LOVE Phase 1! I return to it often when I feel the cravings have returned having cheated too much and too often! After a couple of days, the cravings are history and I feel on a natural high. Phase 1 works best for me when I omit the rice and just have three fat meals. I tend to have bacon and eggs for breakfast, followed by lunches and dinners of some meat/fish with vegetables (my favourites are roasted Mediterranean vegetables). The simplicity of this removes ambiguity for me and keeps me on the straight and narrow. I find I know exactly when I am hungry and I tend to sleep really well on this phase. I often stay on this type of Phase 1 just to get back to my "natural weight".' *Sian*

'Better eyesight, clearer head, brighter skin/eyes, hereditary dark circles very much diminished, skin much less oily, colour in my cheeks without make-up or walking out in the cold, I don't have to keep clearing my throat and nose and I don't want carbs or sugar. I just feel more energetic and LIVELY. Oh, and I'm around 7lb down in about 10 days. Diet, what diet??' *the dark kight*

PHASE 1 TIPS FROM OUR HARCOMBE FANS

The Harcombe fans have come up with some brilliant tips for Phase 1. The three main themes are:

1 Anticipate and manage sugar and caffeine withdrawal

2 Plan, plan, plan! Get ready for Phase 1 and be prepared for the new way of eating

3 Rethink everything you think you know about diet and nutrition

They have also come up with some great tips on other topics, but let's get their tips for the top three themes first:

1 Anticipate and manage sugar and caffeine withdrawal

'Start cutting sugar and caffeine out of your diet now, even if you're not planning to start Phase 1 straight away.' *Kate*

'Drink lots and lots of water, it can ease hunger symptoms as well as help detoxing.' *Lizzi*

'Breaking the sugar habit, that is the most important point. I have thoroughly detoxed and done Phase 1 for longer periods, but if I have a drink of alcohol or something with sugar, even if it is hidden in food, my cravings are back with a bang!' *Johnnie*

'Try to wean yourself off any caffeine habit before you start so you've one less thing to worry about.' *Mamie*

2 Plan, plan, plan! Get ready for Phase 1 and be prepared for the new way of eating

'Plan your meals and prepare as much as you can in advance. Have cold meats and hard-boiled eggs ready for when the munchies strike.' *Kate*

'Be prepared. Work out your five day menu and get everything in before you start. You will get hungry so make sure you eat enough at each meal. Read the book again and again. I found that the more I understood why I was eating this way, the more determined I was to stick with it!' *Lizzi*

'Planning is key. If you don't have the food in the house, you are more likely to find an easier option.' *Josie*

'My top tip for Phase 1 is to clean out your cupboards of all sugary temptations. You'll also be doing your family a favour.' *Priscilla*

'Plan ahead. Fill your fridge with all the foods you can eat and have that wonderful moment each time you open the door when you're feeling peckish and realise that you can eat ANYTHING that is in view and as much of it as you want. Fill the fridge or freezer with a selection of the meats that you love and write yourself a menu plan for the week ahead so you know exactly what you are going to eat and there's no "hungry grab at anything" moments to fight.' *Sue15cat*

3 Rethink everything you think you know about diet and nutrition

'My top tip would be to try to unlearn the years of restricted dieting rules and read the book again and again and again. I don't think I put it down for about a month. It helped me keep strong, knowing I was never, ever going to "diet" again. This is an eating plan for the rest of my life. It's wonderful eating real, honest to goodness food all day, every day.' *Esther*

'Forget everything you think you know about dieting and what's "healthy". Take a leap of faith, trust the rules and don't let your own inner doubting Thomas scupper your success.' *Mamie*

'Research, research, research! Smash the food myths as early on as possible. For many folks, this diet will be a "reboot" to everything you thought you knew about nutrition. It's therefore extremely important that you gain a good understanding of the basics, for example macronutrients, carbs and fat in particular, and build confidence. The five-a-day, low-fat, exercise mantras were so ingrained in me that it was over three months of the diet before I really started to embrace fats, lard and dripping in particular. The sooner you do this, the faster the results will be.' *Howie*

'Don't be afraid of fat! It fills you up for longer.' *Alix*

Words of wisdom from those who've been there

'Don't be afraid of making mistakes! And, when you do, don't panic and don't beat yourself up over it. We learn from our mistakes and Harcombe is amazingly forgiving. You may not "know" it all at once . . . sometimes the "light bulb" moments will come much further along. Always keep in mind that this is for life and you are embarking on a journey that will not only give you your health and confidence back, it will also teach you loads about yourself.' *Virginia*

'Be kind to yourself. If you fall off the wagon, don't beat yourself up, give up and say sod it – pick yourself up and get straight back to it with your next meal. We all fail occasionally – we are only human after all.' *Josie*

'Don't keep putting it off. Tomorrow never comes and what is five days compared to the rest of your life? Be prepared to feel a bit under the weather, but know it will pass, you will survive – we all do – and if you feel ill, it just shows how much you need to detox. Find something else to look forward to – a new book, a manicure, etc. I taught myself to crochet in the evenings – it kept my hands busy and out of the biscuit tin!' *Sue H*

'"I can't give this up" is just a lousy excuse for "I don't want to give this up!" It is only five days. "I'm not prepared to drink tea/coffee without milk." Drink water! It's only five days! Five days is a very short period of time to help set you up for a lifetime of healthy eating!' *Mat*

'Ignore all those well-meaning people that tell you you're doing the wrong thing. They're welcome to all their diety-low-fat-sugary-insipid-junk food!' *Woofighter*

Other practical tips

'Don't have something just because it's part of the "diet". If you don't like NLY [natural live yoghurt] or porridge without sugar, then don't have them. Have things you enjoy eating.' *Kate*

'Always carry a couple of decaf tea bags and/or some fruit/ peppermint tea bags!' *Sue (2nd-Alto)*

'Listen to Zoë's podcasts or watch her videos on YouTube and take one day at a time.' *Kathryn1971x*

'Don't feel that you have to have "breakfast" foods for breakfast. If you don't want bacon and eggs or porridge, for example, try heating up last night's leftovers. Curry for breakfast is one of the best things I ever tried!' *Alix*

'It's OK to eat out if you have to, you just need to be focused. Just speak really nicely to the server and explain you are on a "restricted food plan" and that there are things you don't eat, and would they mind helping you adapt the menu a little. People always say yes. In the first five weeks on The Harcombe Diet, I had 35 meals "out of home". Without exception, each time I was pleasantly assertive with the waiting staff and managed to get Harcombe-friendly meals by asking for help in a reasonable and matter-of-fact manner. A smile helps, of course. In that five weeks, I lost 1 stone and 2lb.' *Lady S*

'My top tip is to keep sparkling water in the fridge. It's refreshing and "fizzy on the tongue" and distracted me from any thought of sweet and juicy stuff as one of the hardest things for me was giving up fruit juice and pop to drink.' *Jans*

'Eat! It's about eating and not starving. There is never any time that there is nothing safe to eat. Eat well at meal times. Don't let people undermine you when they see you eating so much. Eat when you are hungry, stop when you have had enough and take the time to REALLY taste the glorious food. Don't be afraid to eat meat. You don't have to only have three ounces anymore! Eat food you enjoy and, within the framework of the plan, there is LOTS to eat. Chickens have legs so we can have snacks!' *Ellie*

'Jump into The Harcombe Diet with both feet – it really is the best thing that will ever happen to you. Revel in all the new flavours that will bounce out at you when they're not hidden by sugar. NOTHING BEATS THE TASTE OF REAL FOOD!!!!' *Woofighter*

PHASE 1 MENU PLANS

So here we go – the diet. All the menu plans that follow have very simple meal options. We don't want to demand culinary expertise from anyone. If you can roast a joint, cook eggs in a few different ways, chop salad, stir-fry or steam vegetables and add a few ingredients together for a vegetarian curry/chilli while the brown rice boils, you're going to be just fine.

Even where there are simple meals, such as an omelette or scrambled eggs, we are going to include a recipe (R) so that everyone knows how to cook the basics. We avoid milk in Phase 1, so the Harcombe recipes for standard egg dishes without using milk are quite useful.

Our experience tells us that lunch is the biggest challenge. Many people are away from home at lunch time at various different workplaces and so we need to make sure that there is an extra simple meal for you to have at lunch. This will usually be something that you take in to work, although many of you working in towns and cities will be able to buy salad boxes from coffee shops and the Express-type supermarkets, which are starting to cater for people who don't want a sandwich at lunch time.

The classic five day Phase 1 plan keeps lunches practical, in case you are at work for the whole of Phase 1. The weekly, repeatable, Phase 1 menu plans (for those of you who should stay on Phase 1 for longer) assume that days one to five are work days and days six and seven are non-work days. You can rearrange the days to suit your own work pattern.

Please also remember that you can swap any meal on the

menu plans for any other meal, provided that you stay within the 'safe grain' allowance. For omnivores, this means only having one carb meal a day and for vegetarians it means two, although you could stretch this to three if you divide your allowance into small portions.

If there is a day that you really like – repeat it. If there is a day that doesn't appeal to you – drop it. This is *not* a rigid calorie counted plan that will only 'work' if you stick to it by the letter. This is a real food, grown-up way of eating to transition you from low-fat processed food consumption to relishing the food that the planet provides for you.

There is one final excuse to overcome. Some people complain that they get bored of steak, brown rice and curry, salmon in butter, frittatas, roast pork and crackling, chef's salad and so on. Here are two counter thoughts:

1 In the early days, I fully accept that these real, highly nutritious foods will hold little interest for you because you are not craving them. What you really want is the bread, muffins, chocolate, crisps and so on to which you are likely addicted, but this is precisely why you cannot have those foods. We must break this addiction. You will get to the point that cherry tomatoes are the sweetest things you have ever tasted and even milk sugar (lactose) tastes rich and creamy. However, you're not there yet, so recognise your lack of interest in real food for what it is – an unhealthy compulsion towards fake food.

2 It may also help to realise what you have likely been eating up until now. Data on flour and sugar consumption confirms that the average British or American person consumes 1130 calories of these two ingredients alone per day.[1] No wonder we have an epidemic of obesity and ill health. Sugar has no vitamins, minerals, essential fats or protein, and flour is nutritionally very poor compared to nutrient-dense meat, fish, eggs and vegetables. If you have been having cereal for breakfast, a muffin mid-morning, a sandwich for lunch, a cereal bar in the afternoon and pasta, pastry or pizza-based dinners, you are one of the average flour and sugar consumers. You may think that you have been having a varied diet, but your diet has been based largely on two ingredients. Your diet going forward will be based on many ingredients, but you may begin to see steak, pork, chicken, turkey, lamb and so on as all the same and think that you are bored with meat. Meanwhile, although you have likely been eating flour and sugar in different forms, it was still flour and sugar. Don't think that you've been having a terrifically varied diet.

THE CLASSIC PHASE 1 FIVE DAY PLAN

DAY 1
Breakfast Bacon and eggs
Lunch Salmon/Tuna Niçoise (R) and natural live yoghurt (NLY)
Dinner Stir-fry vegetables with meat strips or tofu (R) and brown rice
Snacks (if needed) NLY, crudités (sticks of carrots, celery, peppers, etc), hard-boiled eggs, extra meat or fish

DAY 2
Breakfast Puffed rice cereal
Lunch Frittata (R) and mixed salad and NLY
Dinner Steak and a mixed grill of vegetables

DAY 3
Breakfast Scrambled eggs (R)
Lunch Brown rice salad & chopped vegetables (R) with meat strips if desired
Dinner Garlic & lemon roast chicken (R) with vegetables and NLY

DAY 4
Breakfast Porridge (made with water)
Lunch Egg salad and NLY
Dinner Pork chops or salmon steaks and a selection of vegetables

DAY 5
Breakfast Omelette – plain or ham (R)
Lunch Chef's salad (R) and NLY
Dinner Rice pasta & tomato sauce (R)

THE VEGETARIAN PHASE 1 FIVE DAY PLAN

DAY 1
Breakfast	Soft-boiled eggs with crudité soldiers
Lunch	Coleslaw (R) and NLY
Dinner	Stir-fry vegetables with tofu (R) and brown rice
Snacks	(if needed) Rest of brown rice allowance, NLY, crudités (sticks of carrots, celery, peppers, etc), hard-boiled eggs

DAY 2
Breakfast	Brown rice cereal
Lunch	Frittata (R) with a mixed salad and NLY
Dinner	Quinoa-stuffed peppers (R)

DAY 3
Breakfast	Scrambled eggs (R)
Lunch	Brown rice salad & chopped vegetables (R)
Dinner	Rice pasta & tomato sauce (R)

DAY 4
Breakfast	Porridge (made with water)
Lunch	Egg salad and NLY
Dinner	Grilled Mediterranean vegetables on a bed of brown rice (R)

DAY 5
Breakfast	Plain omelette (R)
Lunch	Tofu & roasted vegetables (R) and NLY
Dinner	Vegetable curry (R) and brown rice

For both the classic and vegetarian menu plans, you may drink as much bottled water (still or sparkling) or tap water as you like during Phase 1. You can drink herbal teas, decaffeinated tea and coffee (no milk, of course).

You may have any soup, free from wheat, sugar and dairy, with any main meal. Lots of options can be found in *The Harcombe Diet: The Recipe Book*.

Replace any meal that you don't like with any other breakfast or main meal from the plan. Have the same breakfast and main meals every day, if this works for you.

THE WEEKLY CLASSIC MENU
FOR THOSE STAYING ON PHASE 1 LONGER

In Phase 2 you will learn what Harcombe followers call 'the no mixing rule'. This is the principle of having a carb/protein-based meal or a fat/protein-based meal, but not mixing the two. All will be explained in Phase 2, but, for those of you staying on Phase 1 longer, we are going to bring in this powerful rule from Phase 2 at this stage. In the menu plans that follow, the no mixing rule has been incorporated so you will no longer be having meat and brown rice together for example.

Don't forget that days one to five have been designed with a 'take to work' lunch in mind. Swap days around if your working week differs.

- -

DAY 1
Breakfast	Bacon and eggs
Lunch	Salmon/Tuna Niçoise (R) and NLY
Dinner	Brown rice and stir-fry vegetables (R)
Snacks	(if needed) NLY, crudités (sticks of carrots, celery, peppers, etc), hard-boiled eggs, extra meat or fish

- -

DAY 2
Breakfast	Puffed rice cereal
Lunch	Frittata (R) with a mixed salad and NLY
Dinner	Roast chicken (R) with vegetables and NLY

- -

DAY 3
Breakfast	Scrambled eggs or Egglet (R)
Lunch	Brown rice salad & chopped vegetables (R)
Dinner	Stir-fry vegetables with meat strips (R)

DAY 4

Breakfast Porridge (made with water)
Lunch Egg salad and NLY
Dinner Pork chops or salmon steaks and a selection of vegetables

DAY 5

Breakfast Plain or ham omelette (R)
Lunch Chef's salad (R) and NLY
Dinner Rice pasta & tomato sauce (R)

DAY 6

Breakfast Rice cereal or porridge (made with water)
Lunch Hot grilled chicken (R) on a bed of salad and NLY
Dinner Steak and a mixed grill of vegetables

DAY 7

Breakfast Harcombe protein shake (R)
Lunch Roast meat (R)* & vegetables
Dinner Vegetable curry (R) and brown rice

* We have three roast chicken recipes, or roast a rib of beef, lamb or a pork joint, as you like.

THE WEEKLY VEGETARIAN MENU
FOR THOSE STAYING ON PHASE 1 LONGER

DAY 1
Breakfast Soft-boiled eggs with crudité soldiers
Lunch Coleslaw (R) and NLY
Dinner Stir-fry vegetables (R) and brown rice
Snacks (if needed) Rest of brown rice allowance, NLY, crudités (sticks of carrots, celery, peppers, etc), hard-boiled eggs

DAY 2
Breakfast Brown rice cereal
Lunch Frittata (R) with a mixed salad and NLY
Dinner Quinoa-stuffed peppers (R)

DAY 3
Breakfast Scrambled eggs or Egglet (R)
Lunch Brown rice salad & chopped vegetables (R)
Dinner Rice pasta & tomato sauce (R)

DAY 4
Breakfast Porridge (made with water)
Lunch Egg salad and NLY
Dinner Grilled Mediterranean vegetables on a bed of brown rice (R)

DAY 5
Breakfast Plain omelette (R)
Lunch Tofu & roasted vegetables (R) and NLY
Dinner Vegetable curry (R) and brown rice

DAY 6

Breakfast	Rice cereal or porridge (made with water)
Lunch	Vegetable egg rolls (R) and NLY
Dinner	Brown rice loaf (R)

DAY 7

Breakfast	Harcombe protein shake (R)
Lunch	Aubergine boats stuffed with rice & vegetables (R)
Dinner	Vegetable chilli (R) and brown rice

PHASE 1 RECIPES

AUBERGINE BOATS STUFFED WITH RICE & VEGETABLES

This is delicious served with the tomato sauce from the Rice pasta & tomato sauce recipe (see page 75).
Serves 2

100g brown rice
2 aubergines
12 black olives, quartered
½ tin chopped tomatoes
2 tablespoons tomato purée
1 teaspoon dried oregano
1 teaspoon dried coriander
Freshly ground black pepper
1 tablespoon olive oil
1 onion, finely chopped
1 clove garlic, peeled and crushed

1 Preheat the oven to 180°C/350°F/gas mark 4.
2 While the oven is warming, cook the brown rice as per the instructions.
3 Cut the aubergines in half. Scoop out the flesh (leaving the shell approximately 1cm thick all the way round) and dice the flesh into approximately 1cm squares. Set aside.
4 Brush a baking tray or ovenproof dish with olive oil and then place the aubergine 'boats' on the tray, pressing them down to flatten the bottom and stabilise them.
5 Pop the aubergine skins in the oven while you prepare the stuffing.
6 Put the olives, tomatoes, tomato purée and herbs in a mixing bowl. Season to taste.

7 Heat the olive oil in a frying pan. Gently fry the onion and garlic for 4–5 minutes, until soft and slightly brown.

8 Add the diced aubergine to the frying pan and cook for a further 4–5 minutes, until this is also soft and slightly brown.

9 Add the fried aubergine, onion and garlic to the mixing bowl and stir thoroughly.

10 When the rice is ready, drain it, rinse with boiling water and stir this thoroughly into the mixture in the mixing bowl.

11 Add the filling from the mixing bowl into the boats and bake for approximately 1 hour, or until the aubergines are soft.

BROWN RICE LOAF

This is a variation on a nut roast. The loaf can be eaten warm as part of a main meal or chilled and eaten cold for a packed lunch or snack.

Serves 4–6

250g brown rice
Olive oil, for frying
1 large onion, finely chopped
2 cloves garlic, finely chopped
1 red pepper, finely chopped
1 courgette, finely diced
1 carrot, grated
1 stick of celery, finely sliced
400g tin of chopped tomatoes
3 teaspoons dried mixed herbs
Freshly ground black pepper
1 egg

1 Preheat the oven to 180°C/350°F/gas mark 4.
2 While the oven is warming, cook the brown rice for half the recommended time on the instructions. When it is part cooked, drain, rinse with boiling water and transfer to a large mixing bowl.
3 Meanwhile, heat a little olive oil in a frying pan and lightly fry the onion and garlic for approximately 5 minutes, until they become transparent. Do not brown. Add the chopped pepper and cook for a further 2 minutes. Add the mixture to the rice in the mixing bowl.
4 Add the diced courgette, carrot and celery to the bowl and mix thoroughly.
5 Stir in the tomatoes and mix in the herbs and ground black pepper.

6 Whisk an egg in a separate bowl, pour it over the mixture and mix thoroughly.

7 Spoon the whole mixture into a loaf pan, pressing the mixture firmly into the pan with the back of a spoon. Cover with some aluminium foil and bake in the oven for 45 minutes.

8 Remove the aluminium foil, turn the oven up to 190°C/375°F/gas mark 5 and bake for a further 30 minutes to brown the top.

Note:

Don't worry about the one egg in this recipe – it is needed to bind the loaf and the amount in each portion is tiny.

BROWN RICE SALAD & CHOPPED VEGETABLES

You can precook the rice to make this a quick and easy lunch time dish. If you do this, make sure that the rice is fully cooked and that you chill it in the fridge immediately after cooking.

Serves 1

50g brown rice
1 tablespoon olive oil
Freshly ground black pepper
Juice of ½ a lemon (optional)
Fresh coriander or basil (optional)

A handful of any of these finely chopped salad ingredients (whatever you have to hand)
Cucumber
Spring onions
Peppers
Celery
Tomatoes

1 Cook the brown rice as per the instructions, rinse with cold water, allow to dry and then chill in the fridge. When needed, transfer to a salad bowl and give a little whisk with a fork to break up the rice.
2 Make the dressing by mixing the oil, pepper and lemon juice, if using, in a small cup and then whisk it into the rice.
3 Mix the chopped salad in with the rice. Garnish with a little fresh coriander or basil if you have some.

CHEF'S SALAD

The concept of the chef's salad is that you are the chef and you put on your salad what you like. The ingredients will vary by season and what you fancy at any particular time. Use this as a time for experimenting, mixing up different salads, toppings and dressings. Here are some ideas to get you started...

Serves 1

For the base
A salad bowl of mixed lettuce leaves
A selection of salad vegetables in season (tomato, cucumber, pepper, beetroot, spring onion, celery, carrot, fennel, etc), chopped into small, but regular-sized, chunks

For the topping (choose
from the following or mix and match)
Hard-boiled eggs
Cold leftover meats, sliced or diced
Tinned or fresh tuna
Tinned sardines

For the dressing (try one of the following)
Olive oil and lemon/lime juice
Straight olive oil
Olive oil and balsamic vinegar (Phase 2)

1 If you are going to have hard-boiled eggs on your salad, then prepare these in tandem with your salad preparation. Place eggs, as desired, in a saucepan of boiling water for 5–10 minutes, depending on how hard you like the yolks.

2 Dice any meat you plan to add to your salad. You can add cheese to your Phase 2 Chef's salad, but not in Phase 1. You may like to add some precooked, now cold, fish or add tinned fish to your creation.
3 Make an attractive 'salad bed' for your meal. If you are having your Chef's salad for a lunch at work option, put the salad in a well-sealed plastic box and add any eggs/meat at lunch time. This will keep the salad as fresh and crunchy as possible.
4 Add dressing to taste. You may like to keep a small bottle of olive oil at work if you have regular salad box options.

COLESLAW

Serves 4

150g natural live yoghurt (NLY)
1 teaspoon Dijon mustard (make sure it's sugar-free)
¼ red cabbage, finely sliced
2 carrots, grated
¼ small celeriac, grated (optional)
½ red onion, very finely chopped
Freshly ground black pepper

1 Mix the NLY and mustard in a mixing bowl (you can leave out the mustard because of its vinegar content if you've been a pickled-food fanatic; however, each serving ends up with a fraction of a teaspoon of something that has got a bit of vinegar in it so it's like the odd ingredient in a stock cube, too small to worry about).
2 Mix the sliced cabbage, grated carrot and celeriac in a separate, large mixing bowl and add the finely chopped onion.
3 Pour the yoghurt and mustard mix over the raw vegetables and mix thoroughly.
4 Season and serve or chill in the fridge and use as required (it should last as long as the use-by date on the NLY).

EGGLET

Serves 1

Large knob of butter
2–3 rashers of bacon, chopped into small bits, or get
bacon off cuts from your butcher (cheaper)
2–4 eggs, depending on how hungry you are
Freshly ground black pepper

Optional ingredients
Chopped red onion and/or peppers
Flakes of tinned tuna
Leftover vegetables, etc

1 Melt the butter in a frying pan and quickly fry the
   bacon, onion, peppers and any other ingredients you
   fancy.
2 Crack the eggs in a bowl and whisk with a fork. Pour
   into the frying pan over the bacon and vegetable
   mixture.
3 Cook on a medium heat until the egg mixture is
   cooked through. Flip the egglet if you prefer it cooked
   on both sides.
4 Transfer to a warm plate and season with freshly
   ground black pepper.

FRITTATA

Serves 2–4

2 courgettes, diced
100g (approximately) broccoli, cut into small florets
25g butter
4 rashers of bacon, diced (or 4 strips of red pepper for
the vegetarian version)
1 small red onion, finely chopped
1 clove garlic, finely chopped
8 eggs
Freshly ground black pepper

1 Part cook the courgette and broccoli, drain and allow
to cool.
2 Melt the butter in a heavy frying pan and lightly fry
the bacon for approximately 5 minutes. Lightly fry the
pepper strips for 1–2 minutes for the vegetarian
frittata.
3 Add the onion and garlic and cook for a further 3–4
minutes, then add the courgette and broccoli. Cook
for a further 3–4 minutes, stirring frequently.
4 Whisk the eggs in a mixing bowl, season with freshly
ground black pepper and pour the mixture over the
ingredients in the frying pan. Cook on a low heat for
about 6–8 minutes, until the egg mixture becomes
firm.
5 Remove from the heat and place under a hot grill until
the top of the frittata starts to brown. Then remove
from the heat and flip over so that the ingredients at
the bottom of the frying pan are on top for serving.
6 Slice like a pizza and serve warm with a mixed salad
or your favourite vegetables.

GRILLED MEDITERRANEAN VEGETABLES ON A BED OF BROWN RICE

Serves 2

100g brown rice
Olive oil, for cooking

300g mixed vegetables (choose from the following)
Aubergines, cut into 2cm cubes
Courgettes, sliced lengthways into quarters
Peppers (red, green, yellow), deseeded and
cut into 2cm chunks
Fennel, quartered
Red onion, cut lengthways into quarters
Large tomato, quartered
Baby whole sweetcorn

1 Cook the brown rice as per the instructions.
2 Meanwhile, lightly oil a roasting dish and spread out
the prepared vegetables on it (if you cook the rice and
the vegetables in parallel, they'll be ready at roughly
the same time). Sprinkle some olive oil over them and
pop them under a hot grill. Grill for 10 minutes, turn
the vegetables and grill for another 10 minutes. Turn
the vegetables for a second time and grill for another
10 minutes. The vegetables should be cooked by now
and starting to brown nicely.
3 Drain and rinse the rice with boiling water and then
arrange in two bowls. Pile the hot vegetables on top
of the rice and serve hot.

HARCOMBE PROTEIN SHAKE

Protein shakes have become increasingly popular of late. The ingredients in bought protein shakes are numerous and many of them are unrecognisable, therefore they don't fall into the real and natural principle of The Harcombe Diet. Here is a recipe for a Phase 1 protein shake, suitable for vegetarians, which you can swap for any breakfast any day.

Serves 2

4 eggs
500ml thick natural live yoghurt (NLY)
2 rounded teaspoons decaf ground coffee (instant)
espresso powder

The speedy method is to put all the ingredients in a blender, mix thoroughly and breakfast will be ready in 1–2 minutes. To make the shake lighter and more voluminous, follow these steps:

1 Separate the egg yolks and whites. Put the yolks in one mixing bowl and the whites in another.
2 Using an electric whisk, beat the egg yolks until they are mixed. Continue whisking for 1–2 minutes until the yolks turn pale yellow.
3 Whisk the egg whites until stiff peaks form.
4 Fold the egg whites into the egg yolk mixture.
5 Gently fold the thick NLY into the mixture.
6 Stir in the coffee powder to your liking.
7 Serve in a glass, like a milkshake, and sprinkle a dash of coffee powder on top.

HOT GRILLED CHICKEN

This dish works equally well with chicken pieces – breasts, legs and thighs – or with a whole roast chicken. Just make the 'sauce' as per the recipe and then smother the chicken with it before roasting.

Serves 4

1 clove garlic, peeled
1 tablespoon cumin seeds
½ teaspoon ground cardamom
1 red chilli, deseeded
2 teaspoons paprika
100g natural live yoghurt (NLY)
4 chicken pieces

1 Put all the ingredients except the chicken in a bowl and blend until smooth.
2 Smother the chicken pieces with the paste and leave it to marinate for 30 minutes, longer if you have the time.
3 Place the chicken pieces on a baking tray and pop under a hot grill for 10 minutes. Then turn the pieces over and grill for a further 10 minutes, or until the juices run clear.

OMELETTE – PLAIN OR HAM

Serves 1

> 2–4 eggs, depending on how hungry you are
> ½ teaspoon dried mixed herbs
> Freshly ground black pepper
> Knob of butter
> 50g ham, chopped (optional)

1 Crack the eggs into a mixing bowl and beat with a fork, or an electric whisk, until fluffy.
2 Add the mixed herbs and some freshly ground black pepper.
3 Melt a knob of butter in a frying pan and add the ham pieces, if using, and whisked eggs.
4 Cook slowly until the mixture becomes firm. You can tilt the pan to move the mixture around to make sure it covers the pan, but don't stir it or you will end up with scrambled eggs.
5 Slide out of the pan and onto a plate (ideally warmed).

QUINOA-STUFFED PEPPERS

Serves 2

100g quinoa
1 litre vegetable stock
4 peppers (red, green or yellow)
1 onion, finely chopped
1 clove garlic, peeled and crushed
1 tablespoon olive oil
1 teaspoon dried mixed herbs
Freshly ground black pepper

1 Preheat the oven to 180°C/350°F/gas mark 4.
2 Cook the quinoa in the vegetable stock for approximately 30 minutes. Using a vegetable stock cube for this is fine – try to find one without sugar, but if you can't, the amount will be so tiny it won't be worth worrying about.
3 Meanwhile, prepare the peppers – making a container for the quinoa mixture to go in. Slice across the top of the peppers, keeping the tops. Fully remove the stalk and 'pithy' bit. Remove all the seeds from inside.
4 Approximately 5 minutes before the quinoa is cooked, gently fry the onion and garlic in the olive oil until soft.
5 Add the herbs and stir in the cooked quinoa. Add some freshly ground black pepper and stuff the mixture into the prepared peppers.
6 Replace the tops on the peppers and place them in an ovenproof dish. Bake for approximately 20–30 minutes until soft to a fork touch.

RICE PASTA & TOMATO SAUCE

Serves 2

2 tablespoons olive oil
1 onion, finely chopped
1 clove garlic, peeled and crushed
1 green pepper, deseeded and chopped
400g tin of chopped tomatoes
A dash of Tabasco sauce
Freshly ground black pepper
100g brown rice pasta

1 Heat the olive oil in a saucepan and add the onion, garlic and green pepper. Cook for approximately 5 minutes, stirring frequently.
2 Pour in the chopped tomatoes and bring to the boil, then reduce to simmer.
3 Stir in a dash, or more to taste, of Tabasco and freshly ground black pepper.
4 Put the lid on the pan and simmer gently for a further 10 minutes – long enough to cook your rice pasta.
5 Spoon the sauce over the rice pasta.

GARLIC & LEMON ROAST CHICKEN

Serves 4

1 chicken
1 onion, quartered
4 cloves garlic, unpeeled
1 lemon, quartered

1 Preheat the oven to 180°C/350°F/gas mark 4.
2 Stuff the chicken with the onion and garlic. Squeeze the lemon juice into the chicken and pop in the remaining rinds.
3 Place breast side down in a roasting dish. Roast for approximately 30 minutes in the moderate oven. This will ensure that the flavours from the onion, garlic and lemon infuse into the breast.
4 Turn the chicken over, so that the breast side is up, and roast for a further hour, or until the juices run clear.
5 Carve or joint the chicken and serve with vegetables or salad.

HERB-CRUSTED ROAST CHICKEN

This is one of the simplest and quickest ways to turn an ordinary chicken into a tasty meal.
Serves 4

1–2 tablespoons dried mixed herbs or a handful of fresh
herbs, finely chopped
1 clove garlic, peeled and crushed
1 chicken

1 Preheat the oven to 180°C/350°F/gas mark 4.
2 Put the herbs in a small mixing bowl, add the crushed garlic and mix together.
3 Rub the herbs into the skin of the chicken, making sure the breast, legs and wings are all well covered.
4 Place breast side up in a roasting dish. Roast in the oven for approximately 1½ hours, or until the juices run clear.

Alternative:
Replace a whole chicken with your favourite chicken pieces – breast, leg or thigh – and grill for about 15 minutes on each side until cooked and the herbs and skin are nicely browned. This is an ideal dish to make in advance and use for lunches and snacks.

LIME & CORIANDER ROAST CHICKEN

This is a delicious and tangy recipe that is perfect for serving cold with a salad, hot with some simple green beans or as a packed lunch.

Serves 4

2 cloves garlic, peeled
1 tablespoon black peppercorns
1 teaspoon coriander seeds
Juice of 1 lime
A handful of fresh coriander, finely chopped
4 chicken pieces

1 Crush the garlic, peppercorns and coriander seeds in a pestle and mortar, then mix in the lime juice and fresh coriander until you have a green, mushy paste.
2 Place the chicken pieces in a dish and rub in the paste. Cover with cling film and leave to marinate for at least 2 hours.
3 Cook using one of the following methods:

- Grill under a hot grill for 10 minutes each side, or until the pieces are completely cooked through.
- Lightly fry in butter for approximately 10 minutes each side until completely cooked.
- Roast in a moderate 180°C/350°F/gas mark 4 oven for approximately 30 minutes, or until the juices run clear.
- Barbecue (our favourite).

SALMON/TUNA NIÇOISE

Serves 2

For the salad
A handful of thin French beans
2 eggs
1 Cos lettuce, chopped
4 tomatoes, quartered
200–400g tinned salmon or tuna, drained (in brine or water, as you like, but fish in oil will 'compete with' the dressing)
8 anchovies (optional)
12 black olives (optional)

For the dressing
50ml extra virgin olive oil
Pinch of salt
Freshly ground black pepper

1 Parboil the French beans, then top and tail them. Hard-boil the eggs, then cut them into quarters.
2 Mix the ingredients for the dressing in a mixing bowl and then toss in the beans, lettuce and tomato. Mix until the salad is well covered with the dressing.
3 Place the salmon or tuna in the middle of the mixed salad and arrange the quartered eggs around the edge of the bowl.
4 Add the anchovies and olives in a decorative manner.
5 Serve immediately.

SCRAMBLED EGGS

Serves 1

2–4 eggs, depending on how hungry you are
Knob of butter

1 Crack the eggs into a mixing bowl and beat with a fork, or an electric whisk, until fluffy.
2 Melt a knob of butter in a frying pan and add the whisked eggs.
3 Continually stir the eggs in the pan (with a wooden spoon) until they become the consistency that you like. The longer you cook them, the firmer they will get.

STIR-FRY VEGETABLES WITH MEAT STRIPS OR TOFU

Stir-frying is a delicious and nutritious way to use up leftover meat and vegetables. You can serve it as a meal on its own, with brown rice, or as an accompanying dish with a main course. Here we have a number of mix-and-match options using vegetables, meats and sauces and a general method taking a 'meat' with a selection of vegetables and adding a sauce. Adjust quantities to suit your particular taste.

Allow approximately 250g vegetables, 150g meat/fish/ tofu and 100ml stock per person

Oil (choose from the following)
Sesame oil
Groundnut oil
Peanut oil

Meat/fish/tofu (can be raw or leftovers) (choose from the following)
Beef, cut into thin strips
Chicken, cut into slices
Lamb, diced into small cubes
Fish, cut into thin slices
Tofu, cut into small cubes

Vegetables (choose from the following)
Carrots, cut into matchsticks
Shallots, finely sliced
Cloves garlic, finely diced
Celery, finely sliced
Green cabbage, shredded or finely sliced
Bok choy, sliced
Mangetout
Green beans
Broccoli, cut into florets
Peas
Courgettes, sliced

Stock (choose from the following)
Chicken stock
Vegetable stock
Water

Herbs and spices (choose from the following)
Red chilli, deseeded and sliced
Fresh ginger, peeled and sliced
Fresh coriander

Sauces (will be used in a tiny quantity)
(choose from the following)
Soy sauce
Fish sauce
Lime juice
Teriyaki sauce

1 Heat a small amount of oil in a large wok and when it's very hot, add the meat, fish or tofu and stir-fry for approximately 2 minutes until lightly browned. Transfer from the wok to a dish and keep warm.
2 Heat a little more oil in the same wok and add the vegetables. Stir-fry for approximately 5 minutes until they start to brown.
3 Add your chosen stock, chilli and ginger, if using, and a dash of your chosen sauce and bring to the boil.
4 Return the cooked meat, fish or tofu to the vegetables and cook on a high heat for a further 1–2 minutes, until the whole stir-fry is piping hot.
5 Serve immediately, sprinkled with some fresh coriander if using.

TOFU & ROASTED VEGETABLES

Serves 4

1kg vegetables suitable for roasting (choose from the following)
Red onions, cut into 2.5cm cubes
Peppers, deseeded and cut into 2.5cm cubes
Courgettes, cut into 2.5cm cubes
Aubergines, cut into 2.5cm cubes
Baby sweetcorn
Butternut squash, peeled and cut into 2.5cm cubes
Beetroot, peeled and cut into 2.5cm cubes
Garlic
Olive oil
250g block of tofu, cut into 1cm cubes
1 small red or green chilli, deseeded and finely chopped

1 Preheat the oven to 190°C/375°F/gas mark 5.
2 Place the vegetables on a baking tray. Sprinkle them with olive oil and then give them a good mix so that the oil covers the vegetables.
3 Roast in the oven for approximately 45 minutes, turning every 15 minutes or so.
4 In a frying pan, heat a little oil and gently fry the tofu cubes until they are lightly browned on all sides. This should take approximately 10 minutes.
5 Toss the chopped chilli into the frying pan and cook for a further 2 minutes, stirring frequently so that the chilli covers the tofu cubes.
6 Remove the vegetables from the oven, give them a good stir, and then spoon the tofu over the vegetables.
7 Return to the oven for a further 15 minutes, then spoon onto hot plates.

VEGETABLE CHILLI

Serves 2

100g brown rice
2 tablespoons olive oil
1 large onion, chopped
2 cloves garlic, finely chopped
1 large carrot, diced
1 stick of celery, chopped
1 green pepper, deseeded and chopped
1 red pepper, deseeded and chopped
1 courgette, diced
400g tin of chopped tomatoes
1 tablespoon dried oregano
2 teaspoons ground cumin
1 tablespoon chilli powder
1 teaspoon black peppercorns, crushed
50g frozen peas

1 Cook the brown rice as per the instructions.
2 Lightly fry the onion, garlic, carrot, celery, peppers and courgette in the olive oil for approximately 10 minutes.
3 Stir in the tomatoes, oregano, cumin, chilli powder and crushed peppercorns and bring to the boil. Turn down the heat and simmer for 15 minutes.
4 Stir in the frozen peas and simmer for a further 15 minutes.
5 Serve hot with brown rice.

VEGETABLE CURRY

Serves 4

Olive oil, for frying
4 cloves garlic, finely chopped
2 large onions, finely chopped
1 red pepper, deseeded and roughly chopped
1 red chilli, deseeded and finely chopped
50g fresh ginger, peeled and roughly chopped
1 tablespoon ground coriander
1 tablespoon ground cumin
1 tablespoon paprika
1 tablespoon turmeric
1 tablespoon garam masala
Salt and freshly ground black pepper
2 x 400g tins of plum tomatoes
150ml water

**1kg green vegetables in season (choose from
the following)**
Courgettes, thickly sliced
Okra (add whole)
Green peppers, deseeded and chopped
Mangetout
French beans
Broccoli, cut into florets

1 In a large saucepan, heat some olive oil and lightly fry
   the garlic and onion for approximately 10 minutes
   until transparent. Do *not* brown.
2 Add the chopped pepper, chilli and ginger and cook for
   a further 5 minutes, then transfer the mixture to a
   bowl.

3 Add a little more oil to the saucepan, add all the spices and seasoning and cook lightly for approximately 5 minutes.

4 Add the onion/garlic/pepper and chilli mix to the spices and mix thoroughly. Add the tins of tomatoes and water. Bring quickly to the boil, then reduce the heat to simmer.

5 At this stage, you can either use the sauce as a chunky one or allow it to cool a bit and blend to a smooth sauce. The sauce can be used immediately or chilled/ frozen for using at some other time. Note that if the sauce is frozen, the spices will intensify in flavour once defrosted.

6 Stir your selection of greens into the sauce, bring quickly back to the boil and then reduce to a simmer. Put the lid on the pan and cook for approximately 10 minutes, until the vegetables are cooked to your liking.

Tip:

If you add 50g creamed coconut from a coconut block after step 4, this will make the curry wonderfully creamy. The tiny amount of creamed coconut that each person ends up with will make negligible difference. Coconut also has anti-Candida properties, so there is an upside.

VEGETABLE EGG ROLLS

The filling for this recipe, refried vegetables, is also known as Bubble & squeak. It is a traditional way of ensuring that no leftover vegetables go to waste. If you don't have leftover vegetables, you can cook some fresh and then refry them. A handy tip is to cook more than is needed at one meal, so that you'll have leftovers for another.

Serves 2

A large knob of butter
4 eggs
Freshly ground black pepper

**Approximately 250g precooked vegetables
(the following work well)**
French beans
Carrots
Cauliflower
Broccoli
Kale
Cabbage
Courgettes

1 Melt the butter in a heavy frying pan and toss in the vegetables, giving them a good stir so that they are well coated in butter.
2 Cook on a gentle heat for approximately 10 minutes, stirring frequently, until the vegetables are warmed through.
3 Transfer to a warm bowl and set aside, keeping warm.
4 Crack the eggs in a bowl and whisk with a fork.
5 Add half the egg mixture to the still warm frying pan (you may need a dash more butter). Swirl the eggs

round to cover the base of the pan. Cook until firm
and then set this aside, flat on a warmed plate,
keeping warm. Repeat with the other half of the egg
mixture to make the second 'wrapping'.

6 Place a filling of refried vegetables onto each egg circle
and wrap up like a spring roll. Season to taste.

PHASE 1 QUESTIONS

Q Why don't I need to worry about mixing fats and carbs in the five day Phase 1?

A Your introduction to Phase 1 may well be tough enough without adding in this Phase 2 rule. The first five days will work well without it so you only need to avoid mixing if you stay on Phase 1 for longer than five days.

Q Why are mushrooms not allowed in Phase 1?

A Mushrooms are avoided for Candida. There is some debate as to whether or not mushrooms do encourage yeast overgrowth, but the early publications on Candida all excluded mushrooms in the recommended diets, so it seems safer to follow this advice. The experts, Trowbridge and Walker and Chaitow and Crook, all advised avoiding mushrooms for as long as Candida symptoms are present, so this is a wise rule to adopt.

Q How do I know if a particular yoghurt is OK?

A We get more questions about yoghurt than any other food. These are the only two things that you need to check to see if the brand you are looking at is suitable. You need to be able to answer yes to both of the following questions:

a Is it live? The pot may say 'live', 'bio', 'contains active cultures' or 'contains lactobacillus'. Any of these will confirm that it is live.

b Does it have 'plain natural yoghurt' written on it and nothing else? If any sugars, 'oses', flavourings are added, put it back on the shelf. If it's just yoghurt and cultures – it's fine ('oses' is the collective term for other forms of sugar: maltose, glucose, dextrose, fructose, etc. Beware the 'oses').

Q Why is natural live yoghurt OK in Phase 1 (if I can't have dairy)?

A Phase 1 came about by looking at the 'perfect diets' for Candida, Food Intolerance and Hypoglycaemia and then trying to design a diet that would be optimal for all three conditions. The diets were very consistent in some areas and differed in others. The compromise I went for, in designing Phase 1, was to allow NLY as it is so beneficial for Candida and there is evidence (see below) that even people with lactose intolerance don't have problems with yoghurt. Add to this that I have seen few clients with lactose intolerance and most with wheat intolerance and you decide that NLY is a very low risk. And it adds so much variety and enjoyment to those tough five days.

> Yoghurt containing live active bacteria is believed to improve lactose digestion for the same reason that probiotics are thought to work. When yoghurt is consumed, bile acids disrupt the cell wall of the bacteria in yoghurt. This releases the enzyme beta-galactosidase (related to lactase) into the intestines, where it can enhance lactose digestion. Not any yoghurt will do. It must contain live active bacteria.
>
> Although yoghurt is a milk product, many people with lactose intolerance do not experience symptoms after eating yoghurt, even the kind that doesn't contain live active bacteria.
>
> *Lactose Intolerance* by Cathy Wong

Q Don't I have to worry about cholesterol?

A Entire books have been written on this topic and I have written tens of thousands of words on it myself. I am one of the growing number of researchers, doctors and academics who believe that the 'war on cholesterol' will go down in history as one of the greatest crimes against humankind. Let's just share some headlines here:

a Cholesterol is utterly life vital. You would die instantly without it. Specifically, cholesterol is vital for the brain, the immune system, digestion, hormone production, reproduction and more. You just need to remember that cholesterol is essential for every single cell in your body and life itself.

b Cholesterol is so critical to life that the body cannot afford to leave it to chance that you will get this substance from food, so the body makes it. Your body is making cholesterol right now. I trust my body to make the cholesterol that it needs and suggest that you may like to do the same. Your needs will change and your cholesterol production will change accordingly. A pregnant woman needs a lot of cholesterol to make a healthy baby, so cholesterol levels should rise on conception. Following an injury, operation or illness, your cholesterol levels should rise so that the body can repair the damage done to cells. At the end of the summer, cholesterol levels should be lower than at the start of the summer (assuming that you sensibly went outside to get some sun directly onto your skin). Sunlight hitting cholesterol in our skin cell membranes turns the cholesterol into vitamin D. So, at the end of the summer you have more vitamin D and lower cholesterol. Don't worry, your body will make plenty more cholesterol as needed.

c Interestingly, the American doctor who started the war on cholesterol, Ancel Keys, declared, 'There's no connection whatsoever between cholesterol in food and cholesterol in blood. And we've known that all along.' Keys spent the 1950s trying to see if cholesterol in food increased the blood cholesterol levels of humans and he concluded that it did not.[2]

What follows is a really important point, which I seem to be alone in having worked out: Only animal foods contain cholesterol. This means that cholesterol in food is only found in meat, fish, eggs and dairy products. To increase cholesterol in the diets of the human 'guinea pigs', Keys had to increase the animal foods in their diet – meat, fish, eggs and dairy products. Doing this had *no* impact on blood cholesterol levels. This means that eating meat, fish, eggs and dairy products has no impact on blood cholesterol levels. End of debate.

So, you can eat meat, fish, eggs and dairy products happily on The Harcombe Diet and have no worries about cholesterol levels, notwithstanding the facts above that (a) cholesterol is vital and (b) your body is making the cholesterol that it needs constantly anyway.

d I could leave it there, but I'll be fair and explain where I think the confusion has come from. After concluding that cholesterol in food had no impact on your blood cholesterol test in the 1950s, Keys was still determined to find a connection between cholesterol and heart disease in some way. He did a study called 'The Seven Countries Study' between 1956 and 1970 where he handpicked seven countries and showed a pattern of sorts between what he called fat intake and heart disease. Keys was heavily criticised for leaving out countries that would have disproven his theory, such as

France, where heart disease is low and fat consumption is high.

This was not the biggest error. Keys classified ice cream and cakes as fats. We know that they are predominantly carbohydrates and entirely processed foods. Keys classified meat and eggs as saturated fats. As we will see in the next question, monounsaturated fat is the main fat in these foods. Keys wrongly labelled food and his conclusions were, therefore, wrong.

This was 50 years ago, so Keys could be forgiven. However, the UK and USA governments make the same mistakes today. The UK government thinks that cakes, biscuits, pastries, ice cream, savoury snacks, confectionery and so on are saturated fats. They are primarily carbohydrates and most of these have more unsaturated than saturated fat (not that unsaturated or saturated is better or worse than any other, but just to set the record straight).

The *Dietary Guidelines for Americans*, 2005 lists ice cream, sherbet, frozen yoghurt, cakes, cookies, quick breads, doughnuts, margarine, sausages, potato chips, corn chips, popcorn and yeast bread as major sources of saturated fats. The Australian Government's 'Measure Up campaign' lists fatty processed meats and baked cereal-based foods such as cakes, pastries and biscuits as sources of saturated fat, so this is not only a UK error.

In summary, you should trust your body to make the cholesterol that you need and not interfere with this process. Even if food can impact cholesterol, firstly, meat, fish, eggs and dairy products have been found 'not guilty' so enjoy these freely and, secondly, the products that could be guilty are the ones that you are not going to eat on The Harcombe Diet (processed foods) so, again, you don't need to worry. If you think that your body is making cholesterol to kill you, you'll worry about anything!

Q Don't I have to worry about fat?

A Hopefully you're feeling more informed already following the answer to the cholesterol question. Real fat in real food is also utterly life vital. This time the body does rely upon you to consume dietary fat, so we must do so.

Fat in food delivers the essential fatty acids, also known as omega-3 and omega-6. When we say that something is 'essential' in nutrition, we mean that it is essential that you consume it. There are many essential things for humans (such as cholesterol and amino acids), but the body can make some of these. The substances that are called 'essential' nutritionally, we must consume. We must consume dietary fat, therefore, and in sufficient quantities to get these essential fatty acids (EFAs). We also need dietary fat to deliver the fat soluble vitamins, A, D, E and K.

Our demonisation of fat is having serious consequences. We are starting to see a re-emergence of rickets in British children. This was a Victorian illness, suffered by children who didn't get enough vitamin D because they lived on bread and couldn't afford butter, eggs and meat. We are now seeing rickets in middle class children in the UK. In 2012, there were two tragic social services cases where parents had been wrongly accused of abusing their children. The children's bones were, in fact, breaking at the slightest knock because of rickets. The parents may have been inadvertently abusing their children, but with the best of intentions – by following current public health advice to avoid the sun (the best source of vitamin D) and to avoid fat in food.

Meat, fish, eggs, dairy products, nuts, seeds and some fruits – avocados and olives – contain fat. This means that nature puts fat in virtually every food that she provides. Just as our body isn't making cholesterol to kill us, nature isn't providing the food that we need to stay alive, while trying to kill us at the same time.

Are pastries, biscuits, cakes, ice cream, savoury snacks, crisps, etc bad for us? I have little doubt. However they are not fats. They are processed carbohydrates and any real fat in any of those foods (eg butter) would be the healthiest part of the product by a margin. It is the sugar, flour and all the ingredients we can't even pronounce in processed foods that we should be worried about.

Q How often should I weigh?

A To weigh or not to weigh, that is the question. Weighing is a psychological minefield and hence the answer to the weighing question is a psychological one. Let's be honest, before we get on the scales we have an expectation. We have either been eating lots of junk and we expect to have put on a few pounds and are just hoping that the scales are not as bad as our worst expectations. Or, if we have been doing really well for a few days, sticking perfectly to our latest diet, we have an expectation that we will have lost weight and we hope that it will be as much as possible.

Weighing is therefore all about our response to expectations and it goes like this: you will either be pleasantly surprised by the reading on the scales (you didn't put on as much as you feared; you lost more than you hoped) or you will be disappointed (you put on as much as, or more than, you feared; you didn't lose as much as you hoped, or even lose at all). Your response to pleased vs disappointed is critical. If, when you are pleased, you see this as an excuse to relax a bit, cheat more, eat more – your success will be short-lived. If, when you are disappointed, you see this as an excuse to give up altogether – you won't get any success next time either. Your mind-set has to be right before you ever weigh yourself:

a If you are pleased, see this as encouragement that you are doing so well and vow to continue to make progress by keeping up your good work.

b If you are disappointed, see this as a sign that you need to keep trying, maybe even try harder, and be more careful to avoid the odd slip. Vow to make sure that there is progress next time.

c If you have the right mind-set, weighing is not going to harm your weight loss attempts. If you have the wrong mind-set, it will.

When you have the right mind-set to weigh, the advice is as follows:

a You only need to weigh once a week and weigh naked, first thing in the morning, before breakfast (you know all this). You don't have to take your rings off and cut your toenails (ha, ha) – we've all been there and it's daft.

b You may like to weigh on day one of Phase 1 and again on day six (after the five days). This should give you great encouragement to carry on with Phase 1 for longer if advised or to move onto Phase 2 if you have little to lose and if Candida is *not* a significant problem for you. We do have some people weighing every day of Phase 1 and, yes, they do lose a few pounds in the first couple of days, but then they get disappointed if they weigh the same on day four as day three, for example. This is not helpful – we need to be patient on our final diet journey.

c You should also be aware of the many things that impact the reading on the scales. I did an experiment in our online support club in October 2009 where I weighed myself every day and recorded the results. The readings varied by 2–3lb (1kg) throughout the month and I consider myself having been at a constant weight since my late twenties. There was one occasion when the reading was the same one day as the day before – likely pure chance.

Just a few of the things that impact weight on a day to day, week to week basis include the time of the month (water retention can cause a few pounds of weight gain for women in the week before a period) and warm weather, which can cause water retention and a few pounds of held water in either gender. However, food and drink in and wee and poo out is probably the single biggest factor behind day to day variations.

The amount of carbohydrate you ate yesterday can have a significant impact on weight on the scales today. Any carbohydrate not used by the body is stored as something called glycogen (runners will be familiar with this term). For every 1g of glycogen stored by the body (and it can store 1lb (450g) of the stuff), 4g of water is also stored. Hence, you could have a serious carb binge and hold 1lb (450g) of stored glucose (glycogen) and 4lb (2kg) of water. This is why you can gain 5lb (2kg) literally overnight. The good news is that you can lose this weight just as quickly as it was gained by having a very low carbohydrate day and forcing the body to use up the stored glycogen.

Q How much do I eat?

A Enough to not feel hungry, but not so much that you feel uncomfortably full. There can be no set rules for this one because every person doing the diet will be different. Men need more fuel than women, taller and larger people need more fuel than smaller and shorter people, active people need more fuel than sedentary people.

Your mind-set until now has been that you need to eat

less to lose weight. The evidence is overwhelming that this doesn't work – you need to eat better. You will be eating calories with a job to do. Fat and protein are needed by the body for everything from cell repair to building bone density. Carbohydrates can be used for energy and that's it. Fat can also be used for energy.

So, when you eat fat, you eat the most versatile macronutrient,* the one that can be used for basal metabolic needs and/or energy. Fat has a great chance of being used up.

On a low calorie diet, you almost certainly eat so much carbohydrate (fruit, cereal, crispbreads, rice cakes, etc) that you have more calories than you need for energy and not enough calories in the form of fat and protein for all the daily jobs that the body must do. That's how you can get fat and sick, while eating so little that you thought you would lose weight.

Try to reconnect with your natural appetite. You should feel nicely peckish before each meal, such that you welcome and enjoy the food when it comes. You should then feel nicely satiated at the end of the meal and for a few hours following. This is about not going hungry. It's not about winning eating competitions.

One particular area of caution concerns fat. Because you will likely live with people who continue to be fat phobic, this doesn't mean that you eat their share of steak fat or pork crackling. Eat what naturally comes with your portion – don't eat everyone else's chicken skin just because you can.

---

* Macronutrients are nutrients that we need in macro (large) quantities. We know the three macronutrients as carbohydrates, fat and protein.

Q Can I have sweeteners in Phase 1?

A Ideally not for two reasons:

a The Harcombe Diet is all about eating real food and embracing natural things provided for us to eat. There is nothing natural about artificial sweeteners, so they don't fit with the essence of the diet.

b We are trying to wean you away from your current sweet tooth, as this will help to stop food cravings. Sweeteners will perpetuate your sweet tooth. Some sweeteners are 80 times sweeter than sugar. If you keep having artificially sweet stuff, you will continue to want artificially sweet stuff – we need to break this habit.

Some people have been such extreme sugar addicts that they do need some short-term help to transition to the natural sweetness of real food. The Harcombe Diet tries to be helpful, practical and workable in such circumstances and we would advise these people to have the most natural sweeteners available, in the smallest amounts that they can tolerate, and to wean themselves off these sweeteners as soon as possible. The most natural sweeteners are FructoOligoSaccharide (shortened to FOS) and Stevia.

Q Can I have caffeine in Phase 1?

A The pure instruction for Phase 1 is to avoid caffeine, but any diet must be workable so it is more important that you adopt this real food way of eating than give up as soon as you see that you should go without caffeine for five days.

If you are currently a high caffeine consumer (five or more caffeine drinks per day) then you may decide to be strict with Phase 1 and give up caffeine altogether. However, a gentler option would be to cut back substantially to one or two caffeine drinks for the first week of the diet, then no more than one for the second week, and then try to cut it out altogether for the duration of Phase 1/Phase 2. If you find that you can't give up caffeine altogether and you need one, or even two, caffeine drinks a day to function normally, it's not the end of the world. Adopting real food is the single most important change for you to embrace.

If you have been having one or just a few caffeine drinks per day, you should be able to give up caffeine for five days with just the expected caffeine withdrawal headache to deal with. If you normally take something for a headache, then your usual tablet should fix this caffeine withdrawal discomfort. If you don't like taking tablets, then you'll need to ride it through. Day 1 will be the worst and it will get better by the day (you will learn how addictive caffeine is by doing this).

Why is it ideal to avoid caffeine? Caffeine is a stimulant. There is some debate as to which hormone it may stimulate. The pancreas releases two hormones, which work in equal and opposite ways to regulate blood glucose levels. There is an argument that says that caffeine causes glucagon to be released, which is the hormone that breaks down glycogen (stored glucose) or body fat to release glucose into the blood stream in anticipation of a fright/flight/fight basic response. The point here is that caffeine shocks the body, as if you had seen a wild animal about to eat you, and the body responds by getting you best prepared to survive. This may be the case and we would likely be quite happy with a 'break down glycogen/body fat' response. However, your body will quickly get used to caffeine – especially if you have a few cups a day – and it will stop getting you ready to fight lions every time you pop into Starbucks! When this happens, caffeine is highly *unlikely* to have a potentially positive impact for weight.

The alternative argument is that the body won't need glucagon to find glucose if there is any in the bloodstream already (and there usually is with consumers of a modern diet). A more typical response to caffeine seems to be that it gives people symptoms of Hypoglycaemia – low blood glucose levels. I know if someone has given me a caffeine coffee when I asked for decaf because my hands are physically shaking within 30 minutes. Glucose may have been released, as the initial response, and then not needed (because there was no lion). Insulin would then need to be released to clear the excess glucose from the bloodstream. Unless this balance was perfectly handled, blood glucose levels could fall lower than normal, so that we suffer signs of Hypoglycaemia.

As caffeine is so often accompanied by sugar or sweeteners, insulin can also be released in response to sweetness and this would further impact blood glucose levels. We don't know precisely what happens with one caffeine drink, let alone several each day, with or without other substances. What we can confidently say is that caffeine impacts blood glucose levels and a key goal in the early stages of The Harcombe Diet is to stabilise blood glucose levels. This will greatly help you to overcome cravings and energy highs and lows that have previously driven you to eat. Caffeine therefore needs to be avoided, or minimised, to stabilise your blood glucose levels.

There is another hormone, which we know is not helped by caffeine in the medium to long term. Cortisol is a stress hormone and the constant stress of the body being hit with such a strong and modern stimulant is really not helpful. Cortisol is strongly implicated in abdominal fat particularly. Hence the potbellied corporate worker who is suffering from daily stress and using caffeine to get through the challenging day. Neither the stress nor the caffeine will help with that waistline.

Q Do I need to exercise to lose weight?

A No, you don't need to exercise to lose weight. Exercise is the 'do more' bit of the 'eat less/do more' theory. Just as we showed in the introduction that eating less doesn't work – the body simply adjusts so that equilibrium is restored and weight is regained – so doing more doesn't work. Gary Taubes shares a very interesting example in his book *Why We Get Fat* where regular runners found that they needed to run more and more each year simply to maintain weight. All the runners in the study tended to get fatter with each passing year. The activity was having no help with weight loss.[3]

Exercise can actually be counterproductive for weight loss. Exercise makes people hungry and hunger is a very difficult driver for humans to resist. If someone spends time in the gym, only to find themselves ravenously hungry at the end of the session, they are highly likely to want to eat more than any energy they have just burned off. Sometimes that hunger can manifest itself as Hypoglycaemia – people can use up glucose so rapidly during intense activity that the body may not be able to regulate blood glucose levels well enough to cope. I have seen people physically shake after a workout and, at that point, they have no choice but to reach for a processed energy gel, drink or bar – and this is not going to help with weight loss.

There is also a pain reward thing going on with exercise. Many people will feel that they deserve a reward after 'being good' and doing some exercise. They can consume more in the muffin in the café in the gym than they used up in the gym itself.

Finally, depending on the intensity of the exercise, food intake may need to be adapted to prepare the body for the session. You will hear long distance runners and cyclists talk about 'carb loading', where they will consume starchy foods, such as pasta, rice, bread, potatoes and so on, before a training session or race. This may help their exercise, but it really won't help their waistline. The individual would be better off from a weight point of view *not* doing the extreme exercise and not having the fattening foods to fuel that session.

Because The Harcombe Diet is all about natural living and eating, we embrace natural activity. Please note the difference between exercise and activity. I use the term exercise to mean something organised and likely unnatural. Activity is the term used to describe living as a human being should. We have evolved to walk, talk, sing, dance, cook, clean and tend the land. We have not evolved to spin on a stationary bike, spend hours on strange co-ordination machines in an artificially lit gym or do a step aerobics class. Such activities are not natural. Do them if you enjoy them, and I mean really enjoy them; don't kid yourself if you don't. If you would happily never see the inside of a gym again, you've started the right diet.

Do embrace natural activity, however. It will use your body and muscles in the way that both were designed to be used. We know that activity helps every part of the body from heart to limbs to mind and mood. Think of that list of natural activities again. Walking is very helpful to get from A to B, but it will also make you feel better in so many other ways. It gets you out in the fresh air, it gives you time to think, it can be visually pleasant – whether walking in a park near where you work, in the countryside or through a bustling shopping area. There are many great reasons for walking – losing weight just happens to *not* be one of them. Similarly cleaning, gardening, DIY – looking after your 'cave' – can all be very rewarding activities. A good spring clean or clear out in the garden may not seem like fun beforehand, but afterwards you will have such a sense of achievement and you'll be aching more than after most aerobics classes. You will have exercised your body in a far more natural and balanced way, and you'll have saved money too.

PHASE 2

THE SUSTAINED WEIGHT LOSS PHASE

EVERYTHING YOU NEED TO KNOW ABOUT PHASE 2

Phase 1 was a mathematical puzzle – what is the perfect diet to overcome the three conditions that cause food cravings? What is allowed in the perfect diet for each condition and what needs to be omitted even for one of the conditions?

Phase 2 is all about reintroducing more foods for the nutrients that they provide, as well as for the enjoyment and variety that they bring back to your diet. Phase 2 forms the basis of how you eat for the rest of your life, so it has to be healthy, practical and effective and it has to keep food as one of the joys of life. I could not sign up to protein-only days or miserable/hungry days, so I don't see why you should either. Such extremes are unnecessary and unworkable. We can't live in this modern world of abundant, delicious food and feel deprived.

Phase 2 has just three rules – that's the perfect number for you to keep in the forefront of your mind as your principles for lifelong healthy eating. I've seen diet books with 20 rules and each of these rules has subrules and the subrules only apply under certain circumstances and so on. This is ridiculous, impossible to remember and unworkable. From now on, you just need to remember these three rules:

1 Don't eat processed foods

2 Don't eat fats and carbohydrates at the same meal

3 Don't eat foods that cause *your* cravings

Let's understand why . . .

1 Don't eat processed foods

If you want to reach your natural weight and stay slim and healthy for life, you must eat food. We shouldn't need to call it real food – manufacturers should have to call their stuff fake food. We have evolved to eat real food. It comes naturally, brimming with vitamins and minerals and nutrients don't need to be added, as they are with fortified fake foods. There are essential fats, complete proteins, 13 vitamins and approximately 16 minerals that are utterly vital for human life and health. Nature puts them all in her food – and in the right proportions and balance with each other. We don't have to worry about making sure that we get, for example, calcium, phosphorus and vitamin D together for bone health – real food does this for us.

How do you know the difference between real and fake food? Think about food in the most natural form in which it comes. Oranges grow on trees; cartons of orange juice don't. Cows graze in a field; Peperami sticks don't. Fish swim in the sea; fish fingers don't. The first in each of these memorable examples is the real food – in its most natural form. The second is the processed food – this is the one to be avoided.

There have been debates about food labels for as long as I have been working in the field of diet and nutrition. All of them are pointless. We don't need traffic lights or Guideline Daily Allowances (GDAs). I have a really simple labelling policy: if something needs a label – don't eat it. Rule 1 makes this your policy now too. Pork, apples, broccoli, salmon, brown rice, tomatoes – none of these need labels. You can see what they are just by looking at them. Don't buy or eat anything that needs a label.

2 Don't eat fats and carbohydrates at the same meal

Now is a good time to introduce rule 2 and then we can combine rules 1 and 2 to give a list of the Phase 2 foods that are allowed on top of all the Phase 1 foods, which you can continue to enjoy freely.

Time for another couple of fact boxes:

Macronutrients – There are three macronutrients. We know them as carbohydrates, protein and fat. All food is carbohydrate, protein or fat or, more typically, a combination of two or three of these.

Foods containing all three macronutrients in good measure are quite rare. They are nuts, seeds and avocados.

Most food is predominantly carbohydrate/protein or fat/protein. Examples of carb/proteins include grains, fruit and vegetables. Examples of fat/proteins include meat and fish.

Don't worry about protein, as protein is in everything from lettuce to bread to fish. The interesting food groups are carb/proteins vs fat/proteins, which we abbreviate to carbs vs fats from now on.

Fats vs Carbs – The best way to remember the difference between a carbohydrate and a fat is that a fat either had a face or comes from something with a face. All meat and fish were animals – with faces. Eggs, butter and cheese all come from animals – with faces. The exceptions are oils like sunflower oil and olive oil (which come from sunflowers and olives), but don't worry about these – the only fats you need to think about are the ones from the faces. Carbs come from the ground and the trees – so grains, potatoes, fruits and vegetables are carbs.

Rule 2 says that you should have a carb meal or a fat meal, but not to mix these two macronutrients at the same meal. This is because of how the body uses food for energy and how it stores food for later on.

Carbohydrates are the easiest macronutrient from which the body can get energy. They start being broken down with salivary enzymes in the mouth and are easily converted into simple sugars for the body to use this glucose for fuel/energy. Protein is the most difficult macronutrient for the body to metabolise (break down) and protein is needed by the body for cell repair and growth. The body will only use protein for energy as a last resort. Fat is the most versatile macronutrient for the body. It can be used for fuel/energy and it can be used for cell repair and other basal metabolic needs.*

When we eat a carbohydrate, the body will use this for energy before anything else. The body would like to store something else for later on (we are hard-wired to store food – our survival has depended upon this). The body will most happily store fat. So, if you eat fat at the same time as carbohydrate, the body has fat available to store.

To store fat the body needs insulin (our fat storing hormone) and insulin is available when we eat carbohydrate. If we eat a ham sandwich, therefore, the body wants to use the bread for energy and store the ham for later on. As the consumption of bread has triggered the

---

* You may have heard of the term 'basal metabolic rate' (BMR). The BMR is the fuel needed by the body to do all the things that keep us alive. We liken it to the situation when you are in bed all day with, say, flu and the fuel that the body needs to keep all your vital organs working, to fight infection, build bone density, repair cells, etc. is your BMR – what the body needs to do even if you are completely inactive.

release of insulin, the ham can be stored for later on. Storing fat is another way of describing weight gain. We do *not* want this to happen. Rule 2 thus makes sure that we have carb meals or fat meals and we don't turn our bodies into perfect fat storage machines.

Put another way, the objective of Rule 2 is to stop the body from storing the fat that we eat as body fat. If you have insulin and dietary fat available, your body can store fat from food as body fat. If you eat carbs you have insulin available, so don't eat fat at the same time.

If you have a fat meal, a few carbs are available from any vegetables and salads that you have with the meal and the body will quickly use these up for immediate energy needs. The body can then use fat from the meal for energy needs. The protein will be the last resort option and any protein will be heading off to meet the basal metabolic needs of the body anyway. As fat can also help with basal metabolic needs, the body will be trying to use the fat from the meal for both energy and cell repair and the fat has a good chance of being used up. Had you eaten carbs at the same time, it would have been a very different story.

If you have a carb meal, there is still protein available to do what the body needs doing. The carb content of your meal is available for your energy needs until the next meal and you've got no fat to store.

Carbs are only of use to the body for energy, so you can see the benefit that fat meals have over carb meals as fats have other jobs to do within the body and have more chance of being used up. Carbs can only be used for energy, so you do need to manage your number of carb meals. If you are having more carb meals than fat meals and your weight loss is stalling, switch the balance to more fat meals than carb meals and you should reboot weight loss.

I have known people come across The Harcombe Diet who are already only eating real food and the introduction of rule 2 has been all that was needed to help them to reach their natural weight and to stay there. It is surprisingly powerful – as you will see.

This is the table of foods that you can add into your diet in Phase 2 with carb meals

Whole Grains	Broad beans	Peach
Barley	Butter beans	Pear
Basmati rice	Chickpeas	Satsuma
Brown pasta*	Flageolet beans	Tangerine
Brown rice	Kidney beans	
Brown rice pasta	Lentils (all colours)	**High-Sugar Fruit**
Buckwheat	Lima beans	Banana
Bulgur wheat	Pinto beans	Date (fresh)
Corn/Polenta	Soybeans	Fig (fresh)
Couscous		Grapes
Millet	**Vegetables**	Guava
Oats	Potatoes	Kiwi fruit
Quinoa	Sweet potatoes	Kumquat
Rye	Yams	Lychees
100% wholemeal		Mango
bread*	**Low-Sugar Fruit**	Melon
100% whole wheat	Apple	Papaya
cereal*	Apricot	Passion fruit
	Cherries	Pineapple
Beans & Pulses	Clementine	Pomegranate
Aduki beans	Grapefruit	Sharon fruit
Black-eyed beans	Nectarine	Tropical fruit
	Orange	

This is the table of foods that you can add into your diet in Phase 2 with meals, as shown

With either meal		With Fat Meals
Low-Fat Dairy	Cranberries	*Dairy Products*
Low-fat milk*	Gooseberries	Cheese
Low-fat yoghurt*	Lemons	Cream
	Limes	Milk
Fruit – Berries	Loganberries	Yoghurt
Blackberries	Raspberries	
Blackcurrants	Strawberries	
Blueberries		

* Please read the section on wheat and dairy (see page 125), as these are the two most common Food Intolerances and the foods that you should be most cautious about reintroducing.

3 Don't eat foods that cause *your* cravings

You crave the foods that feed Candida, Food Intolerance and Hypoglycaemia and those three conditions then lead to more food cravings. You have to break out of this vicious cycle and stop eating the foods that you crave. This then helps you get rid of these conditions and you get into a positive cycle of improvement. Remember that you have to stop the cravings to stop overeating. So rule 3 means:

CANDIDA If you have a problem with Candida (you will know this from the questionnaire and from how ill you felt during Phase 1), then you will need to add the following into your Phase 2 rules:

- Limit yourself to no more than one to two pieces of fruit, on occasions (not every day) for the first few weeks in Phase 2 – this will restrict even fruit sugar

- Stay off wheat, particularly for the first few weeks of Phase 2
- Eat beans, pulses, brown rice and quinoa in moderation (no more than one portion a day)
- Continue to avoid vinegar and pickled foods

Candida is the toughest of the three conditions to overcome and, therefore, it has the most restricted diet to cure it. As soon as you get to the point that your Candida is well under control (redo the questionnaire as a test), you can start eating more of the foods allowed in Phase 2 and eat dairy products, fruit and wholemeal grains more freely.

FOOD INTOLERANCE The foods to which you most likely had Food Intolerance were the ones that you craved before Phase 1 and felt that you couldn't live without. Please don't be in a rush to reintroduce these. If you were a bread monster, the longer you can stay away from bread, the more successful you will be in losing weight and gaining health.

The way to test if you are intolerant to something is to try foods that you suspect are a problem *on their own* immediately after doing Phase 1.

If you eat wheat on its own for example (as plain shredded wheat cereal) after avoiding it for five days, you should have a pretty rapid reaction telling you whether or not it is OK for you. If you have a return of any of the symptoms that you used to suffer from (bloating, upset stomach, headaches, for example) then you will know that this is one of your problem foods and you need to avoid it for some time – until you can repeat the test and *not* suffer problems.

If you suspect milk, have a glass of milk on its own and see what happens. The diet for Food Intolerance is quite simple – avoid any food causing you problems. After a few weeks of avoiding the food, try it on its own and if the symptoms return, you are not ready to reintroduce it. If there are no symptoms, then you can eat it again, but don't have too much or have it too often or the intolerance will return.

Food Intolerances do change over time, so you should find that you can reintroduce your problem foods in the future provided that you don't return to having too much of them on a regular basis.

HYPOGLYCAEMIA Hypoglycaemia is all about things that impact blood glucose levels. Here's an incredible factoid – we need 0.8–1.1g of glucose per litre of blood. The average human has approximately 5 litres of blood, so we need 4–5.5g of glucose in our bloodstream at any one time. That's *one teaspoon*! A large apple has five times the maximum level of sugar that we need in the bloodstream at any one time. All carbohydrates break down into their simplest form of sugar once in the body (glucose, fructose and a lesser known sugar called galactose). If you have recognised that you suffer from the blood glucose highs and lows of Hypoglycaemia, and the energy surges and crashes that accompany this, you will need to manage your overall carbohydrate intake more carefully in Phase 2.

Managing Hypoglycaemia is very individual – it's like a diabetic managing their diabetes. Everyone's carbohydrate tolerance is different and even within an individual, it can vary from one day to the next. The blood glucose mechanism in the body operates within a narrow margin and we have treated it with contempt for far too long by telling people to base their meals on starchy foods.

If you are still experiencing the blood glucose symptoms in the conditions questionnaire (see page 25), the less carbohydrate you can eat, the better. Unless exceptionally carbohydrate sensitive, you should be able to eat vegetables and salads freely, but the less starchy carbohydrate you can eat the better. This means that whole grains, starchy vegetables and fruit will need to be avoided, or managed carefully, if you are to keep the condition Hypoglycaemia under control.

Because carbohydrate tolerance is so individual, you will need to be diligent to see what is the best intake of carbohydrate for you personally. If porridge for breakfast keeps you nicely full until lunch time, great. If, instead, you have a sugar high after breakfast and then a low before lunch, you'll be better off with a fat breakfast.

If you do suffer from Hypoglycaemia, if you have fruit, avoid the high-sugar fruits (listed in the table on page 114) and don't eat more than one to two portions of even low-sugar fruit on occasions (not every day).

If you have more than one condition, you will need to follow the advice for all the conditions that affect you. This will restrict the foods that you can eat, but this is only until your immune system recovers and your body can tolerate your problem foods again. You are not giving up these foods for ever.

Take care not to reintroduce too many different things, too quickly. This is the top tip from Harcombe fans for Phase 2 – they've been there and know that staying in control of cravings is key. If you have any doubt, err on the side of caution and reintroduce foods one at a time, allowing time to observe if you have any adverse reactions before adding something else back in. If you can't wait to reintroduce something, alarm bells should ring straight away. You most want what you crave and these are the things feeding the three conditions. If you can't wait to return to, say, bread, then bread is what you need to avoid. We crave things that feed our cravings. We must break the cycle and then we can return to most foods safely in time when health and balance have been restored.

PHASE 2 PERSONAL EXPERIENCES

My experience with Phase 2

On reflection, I should have stayed on Phase 1 longer. I had severe Candida overgrowth and this took longer to get under control than I had anticipated. My main problem was that I was a fruit addict and so I wanted to get back to fruit as soon as possible.

A lesson to share therefore is to be very careful of any food that you can't wait to reintroduce. This is almost certainly a food that you do need to avoid for a longer period of time.

Phase 2 was also quite a challenge, as a vegetarian with severe Candida, as the perfect diet to overcome Candida comprises meat, fish, eggs, vegetables, salads and natural live yoghurt, with a small portion of brown rice, and I had chosen not to eat the main staples in this programme – meat and fish.

It therefore took me much longer to overcome Candida than it could and should have done. Since Candida comes with cravings for foods that feed Candida, this has the double whammy effect of perpetuating the desire for the very foods that one should be avoiding. Looking back, I just made it more difficult for myself than I needed to.

I reintroduced too much fruit, too quickly, and this really didn't help either. It was so difficult to change my mind-set – I was convinced that fruit was just about the healthiest food on the planet, as so many public health advisors try to tell us. However, the truth is far from this. Fruit is essentially sugar with some vitamin C. There are 13 vitamins and approximately

16 minerals that we need to consume in our diet. Fruit is quite good for vitamin C (not as good as vegetables), but it is incomparable with meat, fish, eggs and dairy products for the other vitamins and minerals. The fruit I was drawn to was not only feeding Candida, but it was causing Hypoglycaemia as well. My blood glucose levels were all over the place during my mid-twenties and I had a fraction of the energy and wellbeing that I enjoy now.

This is my biggest learning from Phase 2: I started to succeed when I stopped trying to lose weight. This is going to sound counterintuitive, so let me explain. When you want to lose weight and come from a background of years of calorie counting, the temptation is always there to eat less. You may be encouraged by a good weigh-in and think 'Great, I'll cut back and lose even more next time.' This just makes you hungry, more prone to cravings and more likely to develop the three conditions. It takes you back to doing what didn't work, though I do understand how ingrained the eat less/do more message is. So I actually stopped weighing myself for many months and put all my effort into one thing and one thing alone – stopping the cravings.

My absolute focus was to overcome food addiction. This meant eating enough and eating the right things to overcome Candida, Food Intolerance and Hypoglycaemia. I had to overcome a fear of cheese (fear of fat in other words) and realise that this was my superfood as a vegetarian – packed with essential fats, complete protein, vitamins and minerals. I had to start seeing eggs cooked in butter as infinitely better for me than rice cakes. Make ending cravings your fundamental goal and the weight loss will naturally follow. Think about it: real food hasn't made you overweight – it's been the processed food that you give in to when you're hungry, and suffering from one or more of the three conditions, which has made you overweight. Overcome the overeating and the weight loss just happens.

Once I got into a pattern with Phase 2, and especially when I made good efforts to reduce my fruit intake, I did find it a pretty perfect diet to follow. I enjoyed porridge with milk for breakfast, a very large cheese salad with olive oil, beetroot, grated carrot and all sorts for lunch, and kept the variety for dinner, as our stock of vegetarian main meals grew steadily.

We reintroduced the 'Sunday bake' in our household, but it was the Sunday bake with a difference: no cakes, no biscuits, just Harcombe recipes that we could enjoy over the following week. It was during this time in Phase 2 that some of our best recipes were created. We would roast a large joint for my husband, Andy, for the coming week and cook some baked potatoes for carb meals for me at the same time. We would do a large curry or chilli or pasta sauce, often a vegetarian version and a meat version cooked alongside. We were then ready for the week ahead and a lunch could be made in 10 minutes by crisping a cooked baked potato in the oven and then adding low-fat cottage cheese or natural live yoghurt and a side salad. Andy could have cold meat, cheese and hard-boiled eggs for a chef's salad. Dinner would be curry sauce with meat for Andy and vegetarian curry with brown rice for me.

Vegetarians on Phase 2 naturally have more carb meals as all carb meals are vegetarian. Andy would sometimes join me on the vegetarian carb meals, but would find the meat 'fat' meals more satiating. Now that I am no longer vegetarian, I agree with him.

Phase 2 is not just the main weight loss phase of The Harcombe Diet, it forms the basis of how you eat for life. Having been in Phase 3 for many years, I still have porridge or eggs for breakfast and cheese/meat or fish salads for lunch. The main difference now is that I have far more fat meals than I did as a vegetarian and, being in Phase 3, I have a lot of 85% cocoa content dark chocolate daily.

Phase 2 has just been the perfect way to eat for me. I can eat any real food, I just avoid processed food. This means I lose weight, keep it off, don't crave anything and feel great. What's not to like? I can eat fruit – just not as much as I used to. I can eat steak and pasta – just not at the same time, and I tend to have rice pasta because wheat just doesn't agree with me. I can have all the foods that the low carb community enjoys and I can have all the things that they don't – porridge, fruit platters, cheese, cappuccinos, dark chocolate and so on. Phase 2 has been the answer to all my dieting prayers and I hope that it will be for you too.

Harcombe fans' experiences with Phase 2

'I originally started The Harcombe Diet for health reasons and didn't even weigh myself at first, but I could tell after just five days on Phase 1 that I had lost weight. People commented straight away about how good I was looking. As the weight fell off me, seemingly with little effort on my part, I really began to relish eating this way. It came easily to me. I enjoyed the food, loved the weight loss and generally felt euphoric. It was as if I'd been set free from all that low-fat nonsense that I'd believed for most of my adult life.'
Mamie

'The Harcombe Diet = confidence. The Harcombe Diet = health. The Harcombe Diet = new, smaller clothes. The Harcombe Diet = choice . . . you're in control of the food you eat. The Harcombe Diet = new job . . . first interview in 12 years and I got it, being more in control, slimmer and confident I went for it, thanks to The Harcombe Diet!!'
RachG

'This is the way I'm going to eat for the rest of my life – it's so liberating to know that! I've got a girly holiday in Turkey next May and am so happy to know I have the tools in my life to be at my current weight even that far in the future, so I'll be the happiest and most confident I've ever been on holiday.' *Carrie*

'Phase 2 came easy to me, thankfully, and the weight dropped off consistently and steadily. I stuck to the rules, loved every minute of it, and still am! Phase 2 has changed my life in so many ways – many more than I thought it would!' *Kay*

'Phase 2 saw me secure a great loss of 56lb in total. I am maintaining this, which is something that I can't say I have ever done on any other diet in the past and, believe me, I have done them all.' *Cazbah*

WE NEED TO TALK ABOUT . . .
WHEAT AND DAIRY

WHEAT

We need to talk about two foods particularly – wheat and dairy products. Since writing my first book in 2004, I have received feedback from so many people who have tried The Harcombe Diet. The most consistent observation that I have made is that modern wheat is not good for humans. Without exception, people lose weight more effectively and feel better when they avoid wheat.

I highly recommend a book called *Wheat Belly* by Dr William Davis, as it explains with comprehensive references how different modern wheat is even to the grains that were introduced to the human diet approximately 10,000 years ago. Remember that 10,000 years is not long in terms of our estimated 3.5 million years of evolution. Even if the original wheat were available today, some humans may not have adapted to it. Davis explains how the modern wheat has mutated to such an extent that it is connected to numerous health conditions. If you are suffering from irritable bowel syndrome (IBS), Crohn's disease, coeliac disease, gluten intolerance, bloating – any kind of digestive disorder – you will likely benefit from avoiding wheat. If you have arthritis or any muscular or joint condition, you will likely benefit from avoiding wheat. Your weight will also likely benefit from avoiding wheat.

The Phase 2 menu plans have been designed to ensure that you avoid wheat, as this has become the most important food to *not* reintroduce. Wheat is the most common Food Intolerance in the Western world and so it is not surprising that it is best avoided. When I see questions from people who have just started Phase 1, asking how quickly they can get back to wholemeal bread, I see bread addicts who need to stay off their fix for longer for this very reason.

It is surprisingly easy to avoid wheat. Oats are not always suitable for those with gluten intolerance, but they can usually be tolerated by people who don't respond well to wheat. This makes oats and puffed rice cereal good breakfast alternatives to the classic wheat-based cereals. (There are very few sugar-free wheat-based cereals anyway, so avoiding wheat doesn't limit our breakfast options that much). Lunch on The Harcombe Diet is not about sandwiches − it's about large salads, with all the nutrients that we need from meat, fish, eggs, dairy foods and salad ingredients, or lunches can feature baked potatoes or oat cakes as the staple carbohydrate. At dinner time, it is easy to avoid wheat. You can still have pasta, just choose rice or corn-based pasta from the gluten-free sections in supermarkets.

DAIRY

The other food to discuss is dairy products. It is interesting to note that wheat and dairy are the two main foods that were only introduced to human diets approximately 10,000 years ago. The foods most recently introduced to human diets are the ones that most frequently cause problems.

Even with the introduction of agriculture and as communities became larger with more animals, giving greater access to milk, there is little evidence that we consumed milk in any significant quantities until within the last century. Although sporadic references to milk, cattle and dairy can be found in literature more than 500 years old, milk and dairy were not regular dietary options until well after the British Agricultural Revolution (this is estimated to have occurred during the hundred years after 1750).

At this stage, we should note the difference between lactose intolerance, a milk allergy and Food Intolerance:

Lactose intolerance

Literally the inability to digest and metabolise lactose – the simple sugar found in milk (and therefore in products deriving from milk). In theory, every human is lactose intolerant beyond the age of about two, as we all lack the enzyme* needed for digestion beyond this age. Only babies and toddlers are naturally able to break down milk as a food structure. This is obviously a critical tool for a baby and infant, as breast milk should ideally be the only, or at least main, food consumed until about the age of two.

Having said that humans lack the enzyme necessary to digest milk beyond the age of two, many children, teenagers and adults are still able to tolerate milk and dairy products. This is probably dictated more by genes, natural immunity and luck than anything else.

The genetic element is crucial. The UK National Health Service (NHS) estimates that 5% of adults in the UK are lactose intolerant, vs approximately 50–80% of people of Hispanic, south Indian, black or Ashkenazi Jewish ethnicity, vs almost 100% of people of American Indian or Asian ethnicity. The United States Department of Health and Human Services confirms this:

'An estimated 30 million to 50 million American adults are lactose intolerant. The pattern of primary lactose intolerance appears to have a genetic component, and specific populations show high levels of intolerance, including approximately: 95% of Asians, 60% to 80% of African Americans and Ashkenazi

---

* An enzyme is a protein (or protein-based molecule) that speeds up a chemical reaction in a living organism. It acts as a catalyst.

Jews, 80% to 100% of American Indians, and 50% to 80% of Hispanics. Lactose intolerance is least common among people of northern European origin, who have a lactose intolerance prevalence of only about 2%.'

Some people will be able to consume milk as teenagers and then develop problems in their twenties. Some will develop the problem later in life. Once lactose intolerant, it is *unlikely* that you will cope well with milk/dairy again, but not impossible. The intolerance could be the result of a temporary immunity problem (due to illness, stress or a lifestyle issue) and your ability to cope with lactose could return.

Milk allergy

This is like a nut or shellfish allergy. It's a lifelong, life threatening condition that must be taken extremely seriously and the substance must not even be accidentally encountered, let alone consumed. It is, thankfully, rare.

Dairy Food Intolerance

The one with which we are most concerned and that is the result of having too many dairy products, too often. We may well have been quite good at digesting lactose, but if we have had too much milk and cheese on a daily basis, the body can get to the point where it is intolerant to the substance – it just can't cope with it any more. This is when we need to give up the substance for a period of time. There is no precise way of knowing for how long. If the overuse has been recent (eg a coffee bar opened at work and you started having milky coffee a few times a day for a few weeks), it may subside relatively quickly. If you've been having milk for breakfast and cheese for lunch every day for as long as you can remember, you may need a longer abstinence period.

If you find that you can't cope with dairy at the moment, you could have either lactose intolerance or what we know as

Food Intolerance. The former is your body saying I can't digest this at the moment (and it may be long term). The latter is your body saying I've had too much of this too often recently and we need to lay off it for a while. You won't necessarily know which it is, but the diagnosis will be clearer when you try to reintroduce dairy products. If you struggle to cope with them again, you've more likely developed full-blown lactose intolerance. If you are able to reintroduce dairy foods, and if you take care not to go the too much/too often route again, you almost certainly had acquired dairy Food Intolerance because of what you had been eating.

If you fall into one of the ethnic groups known to be highly likely to be lactose intolerant, you should seriously consider avoiding dairy products for the rest of your life. The statistics are too overwhelming: intolerance is virtually certain. If you are *not* in a high-risk group, but any of the following apply, you should stay off dairy products until these statements no longer apply:

1 You know that you are lactose intolerant. If you get an acid reflux type response in your throat, a clear stomach gurgling or other reaction when you have dairy, your body is trying to warn you off it. Heed the warning.

2 You know that you are dairy intolerant at the moment, ie, being honest, you've had too much of it too often recently.

3 You stopped losing weight or started gaining weight when you reintroduced dairy products.

4 You find that you crave dairy, miss it if you don't have it and have a tendency to overeat it.

If none of these apply to you then there are good reasons to reintroduce dairy products:

1 They are highly nutritious and excellent sources of the bone nutrients: calcium, phosphorus and vitamin D.

2 They add enjoyment and versatility to the diet.

3 They are very important for vegetarians to reintroduce as soon as it is safe to do so, to ensure adequate nutrition.

Dairy products simply have too many nutrients, which humans need, for me to believe that we were *not* intended to consume them.

Please finally note that even if you don't have dairy Food Intolerance, dairy products have a measurable carbohydrate content (milk being higher than hard cheese) and therefore these foods are riskier from a weight perspective than meat or fish.

Remember that you always have choices with The Harcombe Diet. If you like dairy more than you dislike the consequences *for you*, you have a choice to make. If you are not losing weight, if you are craving milk and cheese, bloating and generally feeling bad on dairy, it should be an easy call to give it up. If you suspect it may be making you hold onto a couple of pounds and you may get a bit of a noisy tummy every now and again, but you love your daily latte, then you'll probably decide to stick with it.

You may like to do your own pros and cons table for what you personally get out of dairy and see which side wins. Sometimes the stress of giving something up is not worth the other health benefits to be gained. I will never adopt a 'Paleo' way of eating because life's pleasures for me include cappuccinos, cheese platters and milky porridge on cold days, curry and brown rice on winter evenings and lots of dark chocolate. Man can live on meat alone and some of you may love this, but I'm not one of them. If you don't have to go that far, see what you can get away with while still meeting your goals.

PHASE 2 TIPS FROM OUR HARCOMBE FANS

The Harcombe fans' tips for Phase 2 fall into three main themes:

1 Don't reintroduce too much too quickly

2 Take your time

3 You need to learn what works best *for you* – it's individual

1 Don't reintroduce too much too quickly

'If there is something that you are really, really desperate for, it's probably best *not* to have it just yet, especially if it's something you used to have a lot of – fruit or cheese. We crave the things to which we are intolerant.' *Kate*

'My main tip for Phase 2 is to introduce new foods gradually. You need to determine if you are intolerant to anything new and if you eat a lot of new things at once, you have no idea which ones are the culprit!' *Lizzi*

2 Take your time

'Phase 2 works best if you take it slowly. Remember this is not a quick fix diet, it's a new way of eating. You'll be eating healthy food and being kind to your body. But depending on your dieting history and how much weight you need to lose, your body may take a while to get used to all this great food. Please give it time. It probably took you months/years to put the weight on, you can't expect to lose it in a few weeks. You may not lose any weight some weeks, don't panic, stick with eating well and it will happen.' *Kate*

'Don't focus just on losing weight, but keep in mind that you are doing yourself good. This is not a quick fix diet, but a fabulous way of eating healthily for life. Good food is better than medicine and it's pointless being thin and ill or unhealthy. Buy the best quality that you can afford as it makes a difference to the taste.' *Ellie*

'Be patient! Weight loss slows on Phase 2 and this can be for a number of reasons: our dieting history comes into play, whether we are cheating, if we are stressing too much about weight loss, weighing too much or overanalysing our food choices rather than just enjoying the wonderful foods we can eat. This is a way of eating for life and our body will let us know when it is ready to ditch the fat stores. All we can do is to create the right environment for it to do so.' *Lizzi*

'Relax! There's no time limit, you have forever to revel in The Harcombe Diet and how good you feel. Your tastes will change over many things, but cravings can still return to bite you if don't keep an eye on them.' *Woofighter*

3 You need to learn what works best *for you* – it's individual

'The balance of fat to carb meals is completely up to you. Some people lose best on all fat meals, some with one carb meal a day. Be prepared that you may have to experiment to find what you can/can't tolerate. We are all different and what works well for somebody else may not work for you.' *Kate*

'Smash your old eating habits. We are creatures of habit, for example Friday-night-end-of-the-week-takeaway . . . weekends agggghhhh. It's so easy to slip into a routine, so to break it I adopted a five-day eating plan. This divorced my eating from traditional seven-day-week eating, leaving me to focus on the non-eating stuff like work etc.' *Howie*

Other motivation tips

'Don't be too hard on yourself. I have spent a lot of months learning about myself and my body, and how it responds to different foods. I was very frustrated early on as I felt I was doing it all wrong, but it was just about finding my own path through. I have learnt not to beat myself up if I "fall off the wagon", as more often than not it was caused by something specific, not me being weak or greedy.' *Sallywags*

'Should you stray, don't give in to the "sod it" mentality and consider the day as destroyed. Get straight back on track and limit the damage. Don't beat yourself up, we are all human. Just try not to slip too often or too much.' *Priscilla*

'Don't panic if you go off track, one slip isn't a disaster, it's what you do next that makes all the difference. Just get straight back on track, try to learn from the experience, be better prepared next time you are in the same situation.' *Kate*

'If you mess up, draw a line under it and start afresh next meal. Try to keep to three meals a day. If you feel hungry, it's a sign that you need to eat more at mealtimes. Don't be afraid to experiment. Buy new cuts of meat, try different veg or cooking methods. Introduce foods slowly. Don't be put off by small gains, they will tell you if foods don't agree with you. Keep focused and remember your body is not a machine. It may have taken years of abuse and clean eating will take a while to be effective.' *Cazbah*

Other practical tips

'If you are feeling particularly hungry one day, just eat as much allowed food as you want. That way, you will not put any weight on and you will not feel guilty afterwards!' *Redfrenchy*

'Definitely stock up on as many different herbs and spices that you can afford. I personally cook most meats using a simple steak seasoning or piri piri seasoning, I even put it into the frying pan when cooking my bacon. Experiment with as many as you can, it helps to (excuse the pun) spice your food up.' *Phil*

'Get friendly with your local butcher . . . they can get some amazingly cheap cuts of meat without any nasties in. Some may even give you free bones to make stocks with or free pork crackling (a great snack).' *Josie*

'Realise that 75% of the supermarket is completely unnecessary processed rubbish. All you need is meat, fish, dairy and vegetables! Just like the olden days . . .' *Jane*

'Plan ahead meals for the day, next few days or week ahead. Bulk cook mince, soup, Bolognese, curries or stews etc for when time is limited so that you always have something in the freezer. If you are out, always have something just in case you can't have a meal: boiled eggs, Wiltshire ham, vine cherry tomatoes, bottled water and sometimes a small bar of 85% can do the job.' *Kathryn1971*

'Address any overeating or emotional issues with food as best you can alongside introducing The Harcombe Diet. It is easy to replace overeating rubbish food with overeating good food, but once you start to introduce cheats, or if you go off the rails, large portions and eating between meals will not help you to get back on track.' *Matisse*

'Make the best choices available at the time within the *The Harcombe Diet* guidelines and get back on track the second you can.

'Celebrate your meals, give them time, they nurture your body and you are worth it.

'NEVER excuse your food choices to others, let them eat what they like and insist that is your right also. You are not judging them, so refuse to accept they have a right to criticise you. Know that not everyone will be thrilled with your success, they just won't, their motivations are none of your business so don't even go there.' *Farrview*

'Don't try to always find a "Harcombe friendly" version of what you currently eat. Start thinking laterally.

'Do spend a morning in the supermarket reading the small print on the labels – you will probably be horrified.

'Don't hanker after things you used to enjoy but are now out of bounds. Enjoy what you can eat now.' *Mamie*

PHASE 2 MENU PLANS

The following seven day plans can be repeated for as long as you need to stay on Phase 2 and should form the basis of lifelong healthy eating in Phase 3 (you'll just have more freedom to cheat in Phase 3).

The classic menu plan for Phase 2 has incorporated the no mixing rule for you, so that you don't have to worry about this. The shaded areas give a quick visual guide to fat meals and the unshaded areas show the carb meals. We have also shown how to have snacks to stick to the no mixing rule – if you are having a fat breakfast and a fat lunch, then any snacks in-between should be fat snacks. If you are having a carb breakfast and a carb lunch, then any snacks in-between should be carb snacks. If you need an afternoon snack, it can match the evening meal planned – whether fat or carb. I cannot stress enough that you will lose weight more quickly and effectively if you avoid snacks. However, the classic Phase 2 menu plan shows you how to integrate snacks if you can't do without them on some days.

This classic Phase 2 menu plan also keeps you away from wheat, as this will maximise your chance of losing weight and feeling great.

Don't forget that days one to five have been designed with a 'take to work' lunch in mind. Swap days around if your working week differs. Remember too that if you like a particular meal or day, repeat it; if you don't like a particular meal or day, swap it for another meal or day. You need to come up with a weekly plan that works for you and just becomes habit – the way you eat without having to think about it.

To increase variety, try swapping in posher recipes for some of the standard meals. There are many in this book and over 200 in *The Harcombe Diet: The Recipe Book*.

THE WEEKLY CLASSIC MENU FOR PHASE 2

DAY 1

Breakfast	Bacon and eggs
Snack	NLY
Lunch	Chef's salad (P1R)
Snack	Piece of low-sugar fruit
Dinner	Brown rice and stir-fry vegetables (P1R)

DAY 2

Breakfast	Porridge with water or low-fat milk
Snack	Piece of low-sugar fruit
Lunch	Oat biscuits and low-fat cottage cheese, celery sticks and fruit
Snack	NLY
Dinner	Roast chicken (P1R) with vegetables and/or salad

DAY 3

Breakfast	NLY and berries
Snack	Cubes of feta cheese and olives
Lunch	Salmon/Tuna Niçoise (P1R)
Snack	Piece of low-sugar fruit
Dinner	Rice pasta & tomato sauce (P1R)

DAY 4

Breakfast	Puffed rice cereal – dry or with low-fat milk
Snack	Piece of low-sugar fruit
Lunch	Brown rice salad & chopped vegetables (P1R)
Snack	NLY
Dinner	Pork or lamb chops with vegetables

DAY 5

Breakfast	Tuna & broccoli frittata (P2R)
Snack	NLY
Lunch	Roast chicken salad
Snack	Piece of low-sugar fruit
Dinner	Vegetable curry (P1R) and brown rice

DAY 6

Breakfast	Fruit platter
Snack	1–2 oat biscuits
Lunch	Baked potato and low-fat cottage cheese or ratatouille
Snack	NLY
Dinner	Steak and a mixed grill of vegetables

DAY 7

Breakfast	Plain, cheese or ham omelette (P1R)
Snack	NLY
Lunch	Roast meat (lamb, beef, pork or chicken) and a selection of vegetables
Snack	Piece of low-sugar fruit
Dinner	Vegetable chilli (P1R) and brown rice

THE WEEKLY VEGETARIAN MENU FOR PHASE 2

DAY 1
Breakfast	Soft-boiled eggs with crudité soldiers
Snack	NLY
Lunch	Cheese & broccoli frittata (P2R) and salad
Snack	Piece of low-sugar fruit
Dinner	Brown rice and stir-fry vegetables (P1R)

DAY 2
Breakfast	Porridge with water or low-fat milk
Snack	Piece of low-sugar fruit
Lunch	Oat biscuits and low-fat cottage cheese, celery sticks and fruit
Snack	NLY
Dinner	Plain or cheese omelette (P1R) and peppers

DAY 3
Breakfast	Scrambled eggs (P1R)
Snack	NLY
Lunch	Cheese salad
Snack	Piece of low-sugar fruit
Dinner	Rice pasta & tomato sauce (P1R)

DAY 4
Breakfast	Puffed rice cereal – dry or with low-fat milk
Snack	Piece of low-sugar fruit
Lunch	Brown rice salad & chopped vegetables (P1R)
Snack	NLY
Dinner	Grilled mozzarella on aubergine (P2R)

DAY 5

Breakfast	NLY and berries
Snack	Cubes of feta cheese and olives
Lunch	Egg salad
Snack	Piece of low-sugar fruit
Dinner	Vegetables curry (P1R) and brown rice

DAY 6

Breakfast	Fruit platter
Snack	1–2 oat biscuits
Lunch	Baked potato and low-fat cottage cheese or ratatouille
Snack	NLY
Dinner	Mediterranean vegetable & mozzarella bake (P2R)

DAY 7

Breakfast	Egglet (R)
Snack	NLY
Lunch	Greek salad and olives
Snack	Piece of low-sugar fruit
Dinner	Vegetable chilli (P1R) and brown rice

PHASE 2 RECIPES

GRILLED MOZZARELLA ON AUBERGINE (POSH CHEESE ON TOAST)

Serves 2

Olive oil
1 large aubergine, sliced lengthways into
1–2cm thick slices
2 large beef tomatoes, thinly sliced
200g mozzarella, thinly sliced
1 teaspoon mixed Italian herbs

1 Preheat the oven to 200°C/400°F/gas mark 6.
2 Lightly brush both sides of the sliced aubergine with olive oil and place on a baking tray. Arrange the sliced tomatoes on the aubergines and cook for 15 minutes.
3 Remove the aubergines from the oven and arrange the mozzarella slices on top of the tomatoes. Lightly sprinkle with the herbs and pop under a hot grill for approximately 5 minutes, until the mozzarella starts to bubble and lightly brown.
4 Serve immediately with a fresh green salad.

MEDITERRANEAN VEGETABLE & MOZZARELLA BAKE

Serves 2

2 large aubergines, chopped into chunks
2 courgettes, sliced
1 green pepper, chopped
½ fennel, chopped
4 tomatoes, quartered
2 teaspoons olive oil
1 large onion, chopped
2 cloves garlic, finely chopped
400g tin of chopped tomatoes
3 teaspoons tomato purée
2 teaspoons dried basil
1 ball of mozzarella (150g), sliced

1 Preheat the oven to 180°C/350°F/gas mark 4.
2 Place the aubergine, courgette, pepper, fennel and quartered tomatoes on a baking tray and roast in the oven for 20 minutes.
3 Heat the olive oil in a frying pan and lightly fry the onion and garlic for 5 minutes, until soft.
4 Add the tin of tomatoes, tomato purée and dried basil and stir thoroughly while bringing to the boil. Lower the heat and simmer for 5 minutes.
5 Transfer the vegetables to a casserole dish and pour the contents of the frying pan over them. Add a topping of sliced mozzarella, put the lid on and pop back in the oven for approximately 30 minutes.
6 The dish will be ready to serve when the cheese is melted.

TUNA & BROCCOLI FRITTATA/CHEESE & BROCCOLI FRITTATA

Frittatas can be served hot or cold and are a great snack to keep in the fridge for a lunch on the go.
Serves 4

A handful of broccoli, cut into small florets
6 eggs
180ml double cream
250g cottage cheese
200g tin of tuna, drained (in brine,
water or oil – as you like)
OR
200g Cheddar cheese, grated

1 Preheat the oven to 190°C/375°F/gas mark 5.
2 Steam the broccoli florets for 4 minutes.
3 Beat the eggs and beat in the cream and cottage cheese.
4 Fold the tuna and broccoli or cheese and broccoli in to the egg and cream mixture.
5 Grease a quiche tin with butter and pour the mixture in.
6 Cook in the oven for 35–40 minutes.
7 Check after 30 minutes – the edges should be golden by this time. If this is the case, turn the oven down to 180°C/350°F/gas mark 4 and cook until the middle is just firmed up.

PHASE 2 QUESTIONS

Q Weight loss stalled as soon as I started Phase 2 – what happened?

A You have almost certainly introduced one, or more, foods, feeding one, or more, of the three conditions. Go back to Phase 1 and then introduce every new food one at a time when you return to Phase 2. Keep a food diary and you'll speed up the process of being able to spot the culprit(s). Food Intolerance symptoms can be immediate (bloating, gurgling tummy, feeling noticeably different after eating) or they can appear over the next 24 hours. If you test wheat, for example, you may have no immediate reaction, but wake up the next day feeling tired and with aching muscles. This is also a classic sign of Food Intolerance. If in doubt, leave it out.

Q Isn't protein the best thing to eat?

A As we learned in an earlier fact box, there are three macronutrients – carbohydrate, protein and fat. Nature rarely puts all three of these in good measure in the same food (nuts, seeds and avocados are the three exceptions). The rest of the time, foods are fat/protein or carb/protein. To eat an unnatural level of protein you need to eat food unnaturally – chicken without the skin or eggs without the yolks, for example. This is unhealthy on a number of levels:

a The chicken skin and egg yolk are the most nutritious parts of those two example foods. Hence, you're leaving the healthiest bit of your food.

b We don't need an excessive amount of protein – as a rule of thumb, the average adult needs 1g of protein per 1kg of body weight. A pregnant woman or athlete/bodybuilder may benefit from doubling this, but we don't need a huge amount.

c Protein metabolism taxes the liver and depletes vitamin A reserves. Excessive protein consumption is not healthy.

d Eating real food means eating food as it comes – not trying to unnaturally separate fat from protein.

Q How can I afford all this meat and fish?

A When you next go to the supermarket, you are going to walk past approximately 80% of the shelves. No more packaged food; no soft drinks; no biscuits, bread, ready meals, cakes, crisps; no branded goods (where you pay for the marketing and advertising costs); no alcohol for a while either. Just think how much you should save.

On The Harcombe Diet all your shopping budget goes on real food – meat, fish, eggs, dairy products, vegetables and salads. You don't give the profitable processed food industry any of your hard-earned cash. Ideally, you will make time to get the best deals from your local butcher, fishmonger and greengrocer and shop the way we used to before we had an obesity epidemic. Shop more regularly to get the bargains of the day.

Yes you can have steak, tuna, asparagus and fresh berries if you can afford them. However, real food does *not* have to be expensive. Own label porridge oats are great value and can be a staple for breakfasts. Eggs are highly versatile 'super foods' – ideal for breakfast, lunch or dinner. Pork comes in many different forms and is a fraction of the price of beef and lamb. Two of the healthiest foods on the planet are among the cheapest: liver and sardines are almost unbeatable nutritionally and in terms of price. If you really are struggling, even having stopped buying all processed food and drink, a more vegetarian version of The Harcombe Diet may be more affordable – more brown rice and oats and less meat and fish, for example.

Q Can I develop new Food Intolerances?

A Yes. Anything that you eat too much of and/or too often you can become intolerant to. You may have rarely eaten eggs, for example, before The Harcombe Diet and now may eat them a lot and often. You could develop an intolerance to them, therefore.

As general health and immunity plays a significant part in Food Intolerance, you should find that the more you eat real food, the healthier you get and the less likely you are to develop new intolerances. If you do find that you are highly susceptible to developing new intolerances, you should follow what is called a rotation diet where you don't have the same food twice more than every three to four days. Monday's staples could be beef, dairy, white fish, lentils, oats and apples/pears, for example. Tuesday could be chicken, oily fish, beans, brown rice and tropical fruits. Wednesday could be any pork product, lamb, chickpeas, couscous and berries and Thursday could be game birds, seafood, eggs, corn/polenta and stone fruits. It is very rare for someone to have to go to these extremes, so just make sure that you don't have the same thing every day if you are worried about developing new intolerances. I've had porridge and dark chocolate virtually every day for years with no problems. Milk is my sensitive food – I deliberately give it up for random days/weeks just to make sure that I don't develop an intolerance to it.

Q If I'm not OK with cow's milk are there alternatives?

A An animal option is always the next best choice – goat's and sheep's milk can be more difficult to find and more expensive, but are worth trying. Next I would recommend almond milk, or rice milk, which are at least derived from natural products and will retain some nutrients as a result. The option I would never recommend is soy(a) milk. There are many health concerns about soy(a), fully captured in the work of Dr Kaayla Daniel[4] – enough to convince me that it should not form part of a human diet. Women of childbearing age should avoid soy(a), especially as we know that it has hormonal impact – evidenced by the soy(a) industry claims for benefits for menopausal women. They can't have it both ways.

Q Is it OK to skip meals in Phase 2?

A Yes. The reason why three regular meals a day is so important in the early stages of the diet is that most people who start eating this way have come from backgrounds of erratic eating – not eating enough or bingeing and starving – and we need to get you back in a stable routine. The sooner your body knows that real, nutritious food is arriving on a regular basis, the sooner it can stop hoarding food in anticipation of famine and start working with you to burn body fat.

Once you have established a positive, healthy pattern, you will be able to skip a meal on occasions. What you don't want to do is to make the skipped meal a pattern or your body will just adjust to it. If you really can't face breakfast, make your three meals a day noonish, 4pmish and 8pmish. However, the sooner you 'break' your 'fast' in the morning, the sooner you will kick start your metabolism and have your body using all the nutrients for the jobs it has to do that day.

The best way to skip meals is when this naturally happens as part of your lifestyle. You're running late one morning – skip breakfast and have a milky decaf coffee out somewhere. You're stuck in a meeting – don't eat the bad lunch provided, just rely on your own fat reserves until dinner. You're late back from work and tired – have a couple of spoons of NLY, to make sure that you're not going to be kept awake with low blood glucose, and then go to bed early.

Q What can I have for work lunches in Phase 2?

A We have put five options in the menu plans. The easiest option is always going to be to take a Tupperware box of salad into work and then something to put on it at lunch time – a tin of fish, tub of cottage cheese, piece of chicken, hard-boiled eggs, sliced cold meats, etc. This is going to be the easiest and healthiest daily option. Add a soup in the winter and the salad can be an all-year-round option.

You may have a baked potato outlet near work. Get a plain potato and add your own tub of low-fat cottage cheese or NLY. Several coffee shops and high street takeaway outlets now do salad boxes for lunch. Some are starting to do no bread 'sandwiches' – such is the power of the low carb movement.

Put a bit of effort into advance preparation and you could have a filling frittata (see page 68) for lunch at work that will keep you going until dinner time. Or prepare the brown rice salad (see page 64). Or bring in oat biscuits and some low-fat cottage cheese. Or make extra for dinner each evening and bring the leftovers into work the next day. There are many options, but you will need to put in slightly more effort than waiting for the sandwich trolley to arrive mid-morning.

OPTIMISING SUCCESS

OVERCOMING THINGS THAT CAN
IMPACT WEIGHT LOSS

When people are losing weight and gaining health on The Harcombe Diet, they don't need much help. They need support and motivation to make sure that they don't slip back to old ways and they love learning new things about diet and nutrition. However, they are generally more likely to be helping others than needing help.

There are, however, a number of things that can hamper weight loss and my experience of working with people over several years has enabled me to come up with 10 steps to work through if you've not lost weight for some time.

1 Natural weight
A celebrity hairdresser I know was doing a makeover and photo shoot for some female cancer survivors and the women were due to be in his London salon all day. There was some downtime for each of the three ladies, while they were waiting for their turn for hair, nails, make-up and so on. I had been asked to schedule a phone call with each of them during the day to help them with any healthy eating questions that they had.

I fully expected the questions to be about optimal eating for health and which foods would be best to avoid to protect against cancer coming back. One of the women, however, wanted weight loss advice. Great, I thought. That's an area where I can help. I went through all the usual 'seeking to understand' questions – What are you eating currently? How often do you eat? Do you have any slips? The answers were role model. The woman was only eating quality, real food, three times a day, no snacking, no cheating. Nothing other than perfect eating was going on. I was really struggling to think how I could help and then I suddenly thought to query, 'Do you mind me asking your current weight and height? Or Body Mass Index (BMI) if you know it?' This is now the first question that I ask. The woman was 5ft 7in (170cm) and had a BMI of barely 19. That's at the bottom end of normal – verging on underweight. I had to steer the conversation away from 'I want to lose weight' to 'how can you accept that you are slim, underweight if anything, and how can you learn to realise that you are no longer the overweight person that you perhaps once were'.

The first question that must be asked, therefore, just to rule out a repeat of this scenario, is height and weight or BMI. BMI is by no means a perfect measure. As a general rule, the taller someone is, the less well it works and it works less well for men than women. As an example, it is relatively easy for a petite person like me (size 2½–3 feet, tiny wrists, etc) to achieve a BMI of 20–21. My husband, Andy, looks fit and healthy, with a totally flat stomach, at a BMI of 27 – officially overweight. Height scales people up overall – there are not many supermodels with size 2½–3 feet. The taller you are, the more likely that your natural weight is going to be at the higher end of the normal BMI range (18.5–24.9 is the normal range), so you are more likely to be in the 21.7–24.9 range than in the 18.5–21.7 range.

When I see people staying at the same weight for a long period of time and that weight is around a BMI of 23–25, I cannot help but think that they are at, or getting close to, natural weight. This is especially the case if the person is male or a taller person of either gender, where we know that a BMI at the lower, or even average, part of the normal range, is unlikely to be natural for that person.

As a general rule, the vast majority of people with a BMI over 30 are *not* at natural weight and should be able to lose more weight over time. When you start getting into the 25–30 range, tall males especially, you may find that you settle naturally somewhere in this 'overweight' range. I would still expect most women to be able to get close to, or into, the normal range, unless they are very tall and 'large' builds for a woman (height, feet and wrist size are good general frame size guides). Taller women in the normal range – especially around 22–24 BMI – may well be at natural weight. This is when we turn to other factors.

2 Medication

It has become increasingly important to consider medication quite early on in an understanding of stalled weight loss. I was shocked writing Chapter Three of *The Obesity Epidemic: What caused it? How can we stop it?* to see just how significant the impact of medication is on weight. Rare is the drug that just so happens to reduce weight. The vast majority seem to be working in the other direction.

You may not be experiencing weight gain, but your medication could well be stopping weight loss. Look on it like this – but for the medication you would be losing weight and but for adopting The Harcombe Diet you would be gaining weight with the medication.

If we try to view this as positively as possible, most medication should be making a relatively small difference to weight. The worst drugs that I reviewed were those taken for serious mind health conditions – Clozapine, for schizophrenia, for example showed an average weight gain of 22lb (9.9kg) over a one year study. Perhaps even more shocking was the average recorded gain of 16lb (7.1kg) in just 12 weeks for Olanzapine for the treatment of psychosis.[5] If you are taking any medication that you think has impacted your weight, you may want to rethink your treatment – ideally working with a sympathetic doctor in doing so. It is not good for you or the doctor if treating one problem generates another (obesity) and they must either review the need for the medication or see if another drug would have less impact on your weight.

You may have taken medication under advice without having been warned about possible weight gain. I sincerely hope not, but I suspect that this has happened to a number of readers. Medical professionals must assume that no one wants to gain weight – women especially – and they must give you clear warnings if medication that they are about to prescribe could result in weight gain or disturb weight loss.

Antidepressants and the pill are two very commonly taken medications and both can cause weight gain or prevent weight loss. However, with these drugs, the weight gain or impact on weight loss should be small – more than half a stone being *unlikely*. If that half a stone means more to you than anything, you need to rethink your medication. If you are able to manage without antidepressants and/or find an alternative contraceptive, then you may like to discuss this with your doctor.

Please also read all medication leaflets carefully and ideally do your own research on the internet before taking anything new. If you do an internet search for the name of your drug and 'side effects' or, better still, the name of your drug and 'weight gain', you will pick up forums where people share their own experiences. Such sites are invaluable.

Take care where a drug is prescribed for a condition when it is best known as a treatment for another condition. I have come across examples of people being given antidepressants for premenstrual syndrome/tension (PMS/PMT), disturbed sleep or anxiety without realising what group of medication they were taking. Such people may be aware that antidepressants are possible factors in weight gain without realising that they have just fallen into this category.

3 Medical conditions

Following medication, one of the most important areas to explore is medical conditions, either those known about or those that may not have been diagnosed as yet. There are a number of medical conditions that can impact weight – the most important ones to mention are:

a Thyroid problems

b Polycystic ovary syndrome (PCOS)

c Diabetes

Interestingly, all three of these significant and relatively common medical conditions (certainly PCOS and diabetes are common) are hormone related. The thyroid gland produces thyroid hormones (amongst other functions). PCOS is absolutely intertwined with hormones, both impacting on and being impacted by hormones from gender hormones to pancreatic hormones. The major hormone in the case of diabetes is insulin, but the other main hormone produced by the pancreas – glucagon – also plays a key part in regulating blood glucose levels.

When someone has weight to lose, has not been losing for a few weeks and there are no medication issues, the next suspect must be a medical condition. Let's have a brief look at these three medical conditions to see if they could be impacting your weight:

a Thyroid problems

The thyroid gland secretes thyroxin, which is critical to metabolism and Basal Metabolic Rate (BMR). We know that the thyroid gland is a clear and definite factor in weight. With no change in calories consumed, we could remove the thyroid gland in a thin person and make them fat. This is an extreme scenario, but an underactive thyroid, also known as hypothyroidism, will lead to a decrease in BMR, weight gain, lethargy and other unpleasant symptoms. Conversely, an overactive thyroid, hyperthyroidism, will lead to an increase in BMR, weight loss, hyperactivity and equally unwelcome symptoms. ('Hypo' always means low and 'hyper' always means high when discussing medical terms.) A blood test for thyroid functioning is one of the first tests done to investigate seemingly inexplicable weight loss or gain.

Funnily enough, I rarely get queries about possible hyperthyroidism. This will likely lead to 'unexplained' weight *loss* and the person will be going to their GP for other reasons. It may sound like the best condition you could ever suffer, but it really is not. The levels of thyroid in the body are so crucial to our entire wellbeing and so delicately balanced that you want the body to be managing this normally. People suffering from hyperthyroidism can feel anxious, jittery, hyped up and just generally unwell for much of the time. I wouldn't wish this on anyone. This is also how someone with hypothyroidism can feel when they first start being given medication for their condition, as it takes a while for the ideal dose to be worked out. (The process of starting thyroid medication is a bit of 'trial and error' in the early stages; the amount really is difficult to balance precisely.)

I can understand that people who are struggling to lose weight may welcome a positive thyroid blood test result (for hypothyroidism), as at least this provides an explanation for weight gain or lack of weight loss. However, please see a negative blood test result as a wonderful thing to receive – you really do not want hypothyroidism. It is a serious condition, very unpleasant and quite difficult to manage. You will be on medication for life and the medication is a poor imitator of the incredible balancing role played by a working thyroid gland. It is very difficult to get the dose just right and patients swing between symptoms of high and low thyroid functioning with all the horrible symptoms that go with this. One day hyped up and jittery and the next day exhausted and sluggish. So, please be thrilled if you get a normal blood test for thyroid functioning.

b Polycystic ovary syndrome (PCOS)

Let's start with some definitions. 'Polycystic ovaries' is literally the condition of having small cysts on the ovaries (usually no bigger than 8mm each). These cysts are egg-containing follicles that have not developed properly. During each menstrual cycle, follicles grow on the ovaries and eggs develop within these follicles. One egg will develop faster than the others and be released into the Fallopian tubes. This is known as ovulation. The remaining follicles naturally degenerate. With polycystic ovaries, the ovaries are larger than normal and the underdeveloped follicles appear in clusters. Polycystic ovaries *per se* are not too problematic. However, they all too often occur in parallel with a hormone imbalance and this is when other conditions appear alongside the polycystic ovaries and this is when we get polycystic ovary syndrome.

Polycystic ovary syndrome is the name for a wider group of conditions – including polycystic ovaries – but also including irregular periods, painful periods, unwelcome hair growth, acne, fatigue, weight gain, etc – all really unpleasant symptoms. Women can have polycystic ovaries without more widespread symptoms, but this is rare. Usually the question is how many of the additional symptoms are present and how bad are they.

The incidence of PCOS is estimated to be approximately 10%, so that's one in ten women of reproductive age. The symptoms often appear soon after puberty and so some women will have lived with this condition for years, if not decades. Many women are unaware that they have PCOS and they may have dismissed early signs of the condition as just teenage acne and assumed longer term weight gain to be something that happens with age. PCOS is generally recognised to be the most common hormonal disorder in women of reproductive age.

The causes of PCOS are not agreed upon. There seems to be a genetic element – a mother having PCOS will be more likely to have a daughter with PCOS. Beyond the genetic element, the key factor in PCOS is hormones, from internal gender hormones being out of balance (oestrogen, testosterone), to glucose handling hormones working less than optimally (insulin, glucagon), to stress hormones being overstimulated (cortisol, adrenalin). Externally, the pill, modern chemicals and modern 'food' are possible factors impacting PCOS. Given the delicate balance that the body is continually trying to achieve, with all parts of the hormone system, I'm actually more surprised that *anyone* manages to achieve balance in our modern world of medication, chemicals and fake foods, not that 10% of women 'fail' to.

The impact of PCOS on weight is well documented and the reasons as to why this would be the case are many and varied. Women who are obese are more likely to have PCOS and women who have PCOS are more likely to be obese. When we explore this 'chicken and egg' scenario, we find that insulin, carbohydrates, glucose and insulin resistance are at the heart of this cyclical problem.

In much of the literature on PCOS, the debate is not just that insulin resistance and PCOS are connected, but that insulin resistance causes PCOS. Here's how this can happen:

- The more carbohydrates we eat, and the more often we eat them, the more likely we are to become insulin resistant. As carbohydrates break down into glucose, the body tries to remove this glucose from the bloodstream and tries to move glucose into cells of the body where they can be used for energy. Insulin resistance describes the situation where cell walls have become desensitised to insulin. So, when glucose tries to get into cells where it is needed for energy, insulin is supposed to assist this process, but where insulin resistance occurs, the process doesn't work properly. The cell then doesn't get the glucose it needs, the body overproduces insulin thinking that more is needed and the person gains weight, with insulin being the fattening hormone.

  When glucose doesn't get into the cells, it is left in the bloodstream, causing raised levels of blood glucose. This is toxic to the body, so it has to find another way to get glucose out of the bloodstream and the glucose is converted to glycogen (stored glucose) and stored in the liver. Within 24 hours, the liver will convert the glucose/glycogen to fat and the person gains weight (and we understand that weight itself makes someone more disposed to having PCOS).

- The second route by which insulin resistance can 'cause' PCOS is that excess insulin (when the body overproduces insulin not realising that the insulin resistance is preventing the insulin already released from being used properly) stimulates ovaries to produce large amounts of testosterone (the male hormone). This alone may prevent the ovaries from releasing an egg each month. Hence, the irregular periods and difficulty conceiving that go with PCOS. High levels of insulin also increase the conversion of androgens (male hormones) to oestrogens (female hormones). This upsets the delicate balance between these two hormone levels and this can also impact weight and prevent normal egg ovulation development, leading to cysts.

The root problem in all of this is carbohydrate. But for the carbohydrate there would be no excess glucose, no need to remove this from the bloodstream, no constant demand on the pancreas for insulin, no likelihood of developing insulin resistance and so on.

The Harcombe Diet is therefore perfect to help with PCOS – real food, with optimal nourishment for optimal health, and managed carbohydrate intake to deal with weight and to reduce the demand upon the body for insulin. We can enjoy carbs on The Harcombe Diet, but PCOS sufferers will need to manage their carb intake even more carefully than the average Harcombe follower because they simply cannot afford to allow insulin resistance to develop any more than it already has.

In parallel, you should try to address non-dietary factors. Is there any alternative to taking the pill? How best can you manage your stress/cortisol levels? How far can you limit your chemical and modern pollution exposure, particularly to things known to impair hormone functioning, such as plastics?

c Diabetes

Type 1 diabetes is the one that teenagers used to get. If you didn't have type 1 diabetes by the age of 20, you were unlikely to get it. We now see middle-aged and older people developing type 1 diabetes, which is astonishing. Type 1 diabetes is effectively the pancreas ceasing to produce insulin at all – the person then needs to inject insulin, or administer insulin in some other way (implants, for example) for life.

Type 2 diabetes used to be the one that older people tended to get. Granny, with a soft spot for cakes and humbugs, might have been the most likely candidate. Over time, her body has had to deal with too much glucose and ceases to manage this effectively as she ages. We are now seeing type 2 diabetes in children – they have had too much carbohydrate, too often (in extreme cases by the age of 10) and their body can no longer remove glucose from the bloodstream as it was designed to do. And still we refuse to change our 'base your meals on starchy foods' dietary advice.

It is difficult to help people with diabetes – type 1 or type 2 – to lose weight because their medication has almost certainly been set by a doctor who is prescribing a high carbohydrate diet, based on what the government calls 'The Eatwell Plate' and what I call 'The Eatbadly Plate'.

Diabetes is a condition of being unable to metabolise glucose optimally. Carbohydrates are the macronutrients that break down into sugars, one of these being glucose. The logic is surely obvious, that diabetics should be told to avoid, as far as possible, the food that they cannot handle – carbohydrates. Instead, we treat diabetics the same as any other citizen of the Western world and tell them to base their meals on starchy foods, substances that break down into the thing that they can't handle – glucose.

I have no doubt whatsoever that diabetics should be consuming real food (they especially have no room for processed food or anything less than optimal nutrition) and substantially restricting carbohydrate intake. However, you will need to find a doctor who will work with you in doing this as medication needs to match carbohydrate intake. Reduce one and your need for the other will reduce (again, surely this would be an obvious goal for any medical professional?).

I can only advise that diabetics work with their doctor to reduce carbohydrate intake and medication at the same time. I cannot advise reducing carbohydrate intake (despite this being absolutely the right thing to do) without a doctor helping to reduce reliance upon medication as well. If someone reduces carbohydrate intake and maintains their level of medication, they will likely 'hypo' (go into a low blood glucose state) as the medication will be trying to remove glucose that isn't there. Carbs and insulin go hand in hand and need to be reduced together.

A likely inhibitor to weight loss occurs when people are slightly, or even more seriously, insulin resistant and have not yet been diagnosed as diabetic (type 2) or insulin resistant, but they effectively are. Fortunately, The Harcombe Diet is the perfect antidote because the quality real food and accompanying nutrients along with the natural low carb intake will help enormously. There will be many people on the border of diabetes, or even slightly over the line, who may never have to be diagnosed with or treated for the condition if they embrace real food/ managed carb early enough.

Because of their carb sensitivity/insulin resistance, such people do find it more difficult to lose weight (the cells just don't accept glucose as easily as they should and therefore the body has a tendency to overproduce insulin), but they can lose weight. It is even more important for this type of person to minimise carb intake. It will seem very unfair that the insulin resistant person may not even be able to cope with much dairy or starchy veg, let alone grains or fruit. However unfair it may be, the pathway to health and natural weight for this person is definitely low carb and lower in carb than the average Harcombe follower can tolerate.

We shouldn't leave this section on conditions without mentioning the menopause. While not strictly a medical condition, it is a life phase that every woman will experience and the male menopause is also a recognised condition. For women, the menopause is a worrying time in terms of weight because we don't often hear of weight loss during the change of life, but we do frequently hear about weight gain.

Menopause literally means 'the end of monthly cycles'. There are many physical, psychological and emotional symptoms characterising the menopause, but the official definition marks the time when a woman stops having periods. The cessation of periods is an indication that the ovaries have stopped their main function of ripening and releasing eggs and releasing hormones that lead to a build-up of the lining of the womb, which is then shed if the eggs are not fertilised. After the menopause, oestrogen continues to be produced in the ovaries and in other areas of the body (in bone and blood vessels). However, oestrogen levels fall substantially post menopause.

To understand why this impacts weight, we need to talk about rats. Experiments with rats have shown that the removal of ovaries (and therefore the hormone oestrogen) can lead to excessive hunger and inactivity (and weight gain).[6] This can be observed in women following the removal of ovaries, as may happen with certain types of hysterectomy or treatment for ovarian cancer. This known impact of reduced oestrogen on appetite and activity can be viewed as an indirect impact on weight. There is also a direct impact.

The Wade and Gray rat study (one of the two studies referenced, see page 257) noted that oestrogen and testosterone tend to decrease adiposity (human fat tissue), while progesterone increases it. A reduction in oestrogen can therefore have a direct impact on weight, and not just an indirect impact through appetite. The progesterone observation is also interesting, as progesterone is the hormone that rises from day 14 of the menstrual cycle, coinciding with noticeable weight gain for many women. Additionally, the most common hormone taken by females, the pill, typically contains 150mg of progesterone and 30mg of oestrogen for the combined pill and 350mg of progesterone for the progesterone only pill (POP). Women taking the pill commonly report weight gain.

So, in what we women know as 'fat week', the week before our period, progesterone is high and oestrogen is low. Oestrogen peaks and progesterone is lowest mid-cycle, around day 14, when most women report feeling at their peak of wellbeing.

4 What happened before?

If you have weight to lose and have ruled out medication or medical conditions for a plateau, the next factor to explore is your weight and dieting history.

To get an insight into our current weight and weight loss, recent history will be very helpful. Have you been overweight since childhood? Have you ever been close to a possible natural weight? Were you slim as a child and then developed a weight problem in adulthood? Was that weight gain linked to circumstances, eg pregnancies/children (they affect parents of both genders, although the mother more)? Was it linked to a particularly difficult job, maybe travelling/high stress? Was illness involved – either for you or someone else in the family?

The key factors to establish are:

a Have you ever been at a possible natural weight?

b If so, how long did you stay at a particular weight?

c When were you last at this weight?

If you have never been at a weight that you found relatively easy to maintain or if it was a long time ago when you were in this situation, weight loss is going to be more difficult for you. If you can recall having quite a stable weight for months or years and this was within the past few years, weight loss is going to be easier for you. If your weight gain was due to circumstances that have now changed (eg having toddlers and being too exhausted to sleep and eat properly), you will find the improved current environment to your benefit. If you are still in the situation that led to weight gain (eg having a stressful job and travelling lots), then you will continue to find your lifestyle *not* conducive to weight loss.

Understanding when weight changed and possible reasons as to why is like gathering evidence in a crime. It helps us to understand timescales, possible causes and therefore likely solutions. A lifelong weight problem is a different challenge to a recent gain for circumstantial reasons. The phrase 'quickly on/quickly off' is a welcome one for many people and a worrying truism for those who have been overweight for as long as they can remember. Because this factor is so individual, it is not possible to make general recommendations. Hopefully, the principles of how recently and for how long you may have been at a natural weight will help you to understand how what has happened before – for you – is impacting your current success.

5 Expectations

When I went on my first calorie controlled diet, at the age of 15, I had the book in my hand that said, 'One pound equals 3500 calories and to lose a pound, you need to create a deficit of 3500 calories.' Hence, I was advised to eat 1000 calories a day and, assuming that I needed 2000, I would lose 7 x 1000 = 2lb (1kg) per week. The first week I lost more than this (less than I did when I first tried Phase 1) and there were some early weeks when I lost 2lb but, in no time at all, I was losing a pound if I was lucky or less than a pound – or even weighing more than the previous week because I had no understanding of natural weight fluctuations at the time.

I starved for over a year, dropping to 300–400 calories for weeks at the height of what had become anorexia. During that time I had gone from approximately 8½ stone (54kg) to under 6 stone (38kg). I should have lost 104lb (47kg) in fat alone – more in lean tissue and water – in the first year. I should have disappeared to no weight at all within that first year, but it just doesn't happen. There is no formula. The cruel expectation that we will consistently lose 2lb per week has no evidence base whatsoever, and yet it is in the minds of most people when they try something that will work – Dukan, Harcombe, Paleo – anything that isn't about calories.

In case you're thinking that my 40lb (18kg) weight loss in approximately 18 months sounds good and that you would/could starve for this length of time to lose 40lb, this is what else happened at the time: cessation of periods; loss of muscle and lean tissue; frequent fainting and physical collapses; and I lost a year of my life when I could think about nothing other than food, weight, calories and scales. I was isolated, dull, obsessed and utterly, utterly miserable.

If that doesn't put you off, what happened next might. The rampant cravings started and, by the age of 17, I had regained all the weight lost and was closer to 10 stone (64kg) by the age of 18. Bulimic, addicted, bloated, full of self loathing and still utterly, utterly miserable, overeating was the equal and opposite reaction to the starvation that I had inflicted on my body.

If any of you have been able to lose weight and keep it off with eating less and/or doing more – you won't be reading this book. You will be a restrained eater for life. Such people will probably be hungry, obsessed and miserable, but they may be OK putting up with this to stay slim in their own addicted, lifelong-deprivation way.

The purpose of sharing this is to remind us that there is no formula. We will not lose 2lb per week or any fixed amount per week, week in, week out. I know that you want to follow a 7lb (3kg) loss in Phase 1 with a steady few pounds a week in Phase 2, and it might happen, but it is more likely that it won't. It will far more likely be erratic, stop/start, with plateaus and sporadic drops – there is no formula.

One thing that needs to be adjusted, therefore, and I hate saying this, but it needs to be said – is expectations. I have had comments from people saying they've lost nothing for ages and then you find out that they've lost a pound one week, and then half a pound, and then nothing, and then another pound and this is 'nothing' in their mind because it hasn't been 2lb a week. I can absolutely guarantee that you *won't* lose 2lb a week, week in, week out, until you become weightless! You may lose 10lb (5kg) the first week, 5lb (2kg) the second week, 0–3lbs (0–1kg) a week for a few weeks, then plateau, then drop 3lb (1kg), then plateau – every person will lose a different amount at a different rate. There is no formula and the diets that promise you that there is are lying.

This section on optimising success is taking us through the factors that we need to consider that could be impacting weight loss, in a considered order. We need to start with natural weight, medication, medical conditions, weight history and expectations, as these are the most important things to understand/rule out before looking into other things that could be impairing weight loss. The first five points in this section have therefore been in a deliberate order.

The next five points can be investigated in any order. Many of them are equal in importance or likelihood. So don't worry as much with the order of the following factors to explore.

6 The conditions

If you have lost well with Phase 1 and then this suddenly stops in Phase 2, it is almost certainly because of something that has been introduced in Phase 2. The chief suspects are always wheat and dairy. If wheat has been reintroduced, we can pretty much stop the search for the culprit. Usually if someone cuts out wheat again and stays off it (opting for rice, couscous, oat and baked potato staple carbs instead), the weight loss will resume. If this doesn't happen, then dairy is the next suspect.

The quickest way to find a possible problem food is as follows. Repeat Phase 1, so that you have ensured that any possible offending foods have cleared your system, and then reintroduce foods one at a time, on their own, allowing time to observe any reactions. Keep a food diary and remember that some reactions are immediate (bloating, rings tight on fingers, ie immediate water retention) and some appear at approximately the 24-hour mark (muscle aches, fatigue, fogginess, etc). If you doubt that wheat is a problem and are determined to test it, then try wheat on its own for one meal (eg shredded wheat for breakfast – no milk). Don't test any other food until the 24 hours is up and then you won't 'muddy the test water'. If you don't think that wheat is a problem, look out for it after a few days because it may build up again quite quickly and you may need to avoid it for longer. If you do go back to wheat, don't have it every day, try to have a number of wheat-free days each week – it's just too risky for intolerance for humans in its current modified form.

The cravings question remains one of the most powerful to identify problem foods: What would you least like to give up? What did you miss most in Phase 1? Be really honest because, sadly, that's what you probably need to give up – at least for a while. I used to have terrible dairy intolerance and now enjoy it a couple of times a day. Wheat, on the other hand, I only have on rare occasions – I get away with it when I do, but I would never push my luck with this one.

7 Cheating?

A sensitive one, which we must tackle at some stage if we rule out the first five factors, is accurate intake. Are you eating/cheating more than you think?

If you haven't been cheating at all and you haven't reintroduced anything to which you are intolerant, you could well be at your natural weight. If my current weight were higher than I felt that it should be, I would rather know that I had been cheating and that this was why I had been gaining/not losing, rather than have to accept that I was at my natural weight.

Keeping a food diary is an absolute necessity if the fundamentals of medication, medical conditions, history and so on have been ruled out. I recommend keeping a 'to the letter' food diary for at least a week and one of two things will happen:

i You will notice things that have been consumed that seemed insignificant, but they're not. Scraps from plates during clearing, a sandwich 'because you were out and about that day', a glass of wine, which turned into a few because it was a special occasion, etc.

OR

ii You have a perfect food diary for the week and lose a pound or two.

If you have a perfect food diary and you are confident that this has been a typical week and you have not lost for several weeks, you could well be at natural weight.

Now is a great time to share a quotation from Sue H:

'Keep a food diary and be honest in it – no one else is going to read it so don't be shy! It's easy to cheat a little and then a little more, but if you're honest with your diary you will see where you're going wrong. I couldn't understand why my weight stalled every time I'd lost 10lb or so until I kept a strict diary. After one such stalling, I looked back over my diary and could see that all my meals were spot on, but I'd had 33 cheats in a 14 day period!! If I hadn't kept the diary, I would never have realised this.'

This brings us nicely on to . . .

8 Plateaus

If you are eating nothing but meat/fish/eggs/veg/salad (most people get back to this core if nothing has been shifting for a few weeks) and you have been doing this for a few weeks and still not had further loss *and* if you have a BMI around 30 or higher – I still don't think that this will be your natural weight.

One of the people I most admire in The Harcombe Diet Club is a beautiful, young maths teacher called Lird. She experienced such a long plateau and never gave up and never lost hope. She had lost well initially and then experienced this very long plateau, with no obvious reason why, but she just stuck to the diet and carried on even when the scales showed no success. Finally, a second phase of weight loss kicked in and Lird is now an absolute stunner and finding it easy to stay at her natural weight.

We know that the body is hard-wired to hold onto fat. We know that it doesn't naturally like losing weight. We also know that the body likes to work optimally and carrying a large amount of excess weight is not optimal or efficient and the body will have good reason to dump this. However, the body doesn't want to lose that last half stone, or even stone, as this is what will see you through the famine that the body always assumes is around the corner. Often you can adjust to the regular healthy meals on The Harcombe Diet quite quickly and we see the body quite happily letting weight go. Some of you may be better survivors and better programmed to store fat and you may be the ones to experience the worst plateaus. We don't know enough by any means about plateaus, but all the experts in the low carb field acknowledge them. Mark Sisson, Dr John Briffa and Jonathan Bailor will all be honest and say that nothing can be predicted and that there will be periods where no weight is lost.

This is the real test of character. I know from my bad eating days that if I got on the scale and I hadn't lost, I would think 'sod it' and vow to eat whatever I wanted that day and start again tomorrow. The following day, I would just have more to lose, more cravings, feel carb bloated and hung over. This was never a good decision to make.

My top tip is this: the sooner that you see The Harcombe Diet as a way of life and not something you go on and then go back to cornflakes for breakfast, sandwiches for lunch and pasta for tea, the sooner you will be in a pattern that will get you to natural weight and optimal health in time.

The decision that finally solved my weight problem was to stop trying to lose weight. I realised that I made bad decisions when I tried to make this my goal. The day I switched my goal to 'I'm going to eat as well as I can and make sure that I don't binge or starve and do everything I can to overcome cravings', was the day that I started to make progress. When you vow to eat well and stay free from cravings, the weight follows. Obsess about weight and the temptation to eat less or eat fruit 'because it must be good for me' is always there.

9 Giving the body reason/opportunity to burn fat

Weight loss is the process whereby the body breaks down a structure called triglyceride. A triglyceride is three fatty acids joined together on a 'backbone' of glycerol. Breaking down triglyceride is what we need to happen for us to lose weight. We know that nothing can force the body to break down fat/lose weight and the body has many defence mechanisms to try to stop this happening. We need to give the body *no* reason *not* to break down fat. That's a subtle and important difference.

If the body has glucose available, it has *no* need to break down fat, hence the power of the not mixing rule. If we have a carb meal, we enable the body to use any of the carbs eaten for fuel and we don't give the body fat to store at the same time. If we have a fat meal, we enable the body to use any of the fat eaten for fuel and there should be little/none left by the time the next meal comes round.

The additional power of fat meals is that fat and protein have 'jobs to do' within the body. Hence our meat/fish/eggs etc eaten at a meal can be used for energy (normal body and brain activity), but they can also be used for all the basal metabolic needs in the body. Hence fat meals can always meet two roles; carb meals are for energy above basal metabolic needs only.

The rules of Phase 2: eating real food, three times a day and avoiding the specific food(s) that have been feeding our own personal cravings, work for most people, most of the time. It naturally sets up the environment where we give the body *no* reason *not* to break down fat.

However, if your weight loss has stalled for some time, we need to look at additional ways to give your body *no* reason *not* to break down fat. Here are my top two tips for this:

i The body will have reason to break down triglyceride (body fat) when no glucose is available *and* when either the brain needs glucose for fuel and/or the body needs glucose/fat for energy. In this circumstance, the body has a need to break down fat and *no* reason *not* to break down fat.

   The two things that you can do to place a demand on fuel, therefore, are to be human. Use your brain – think, read, try to have a mentally challenging job or hobby

– the demand for glucose from the brain can be increased in this way. Use your body – move naturally as a human being would in natural circumstances. Walking really is the most wonderful activity – relaxing, stress busting, functional, cheap and enjoyed by dogs. Walk to get from A to B where possible rather than using lifts or escalators or cars for short distances. I can't get over the fact that in our village of 75 houses, where no house is further than 5 minutes' walk to the centre of the village, most of the mums drive to the centre for the school bus. Walk, wash up, clean the house, do some gardening, if you are fortunate enough to have a garden, and dance. Be naturally human to give the body some reason to break down fat.

ii Try something called intermittent fasting. If the body has an occasional missed meal, especially where this can naturally be achieved in your lifestyle, eg if you had a hectic day at work and just happened to miss lunch, then it, again, has *no* reason *not* to break down fat.

To avoid confusion, one of the most important rules in The Harcombe Diet is to eat three meals a day. Most of us have had such erratic eating in the past (bingeing and starving or grazing on low-fat foods all day long) that it is really important to re-establish regular eating patterns. The body likes to know that it is getting regular fuel and it will use that fuel more effectively when it isn't storing everything that comes in because it doesn't know when the next meal may be.

I am *not* encouraging you to skip meals regularly, but I am saying that the odd meal missed, as part of a natural lifestyle, may be helpful if your weight loss has stalled. It will give your body *no* reason *not* to burn body fat.

I have been asked, 'I'm going on a long flight, how can I

manage when I know that the aeroplane food is going to be unsuitable?' In the nicest possible way, I need to point out that even a slim person has a good 20lb (10kg) of fat to fall back on. Obese people have many multiples of this. We are not going to die even if we don't eat for 24–36 hours. Wouldn't it be great to lose a couple of pounds on a trip between London and Sydney? If the food on the plane isn't suitable, don't eat it. If you're stuck in a meeting at work and only sandwiches are on offer, don't eat them. See any event like this as an opportunity to lose weight – to give your body *no* reason *not* to burn fat.

The secret to being able to skip a meal is to have stable blood glucose levels. If you are in a state of low blood glucose (Hypoglycaemia), your body will be doing everything that it can to make you eat, to overcome what it perceives as a dangerous situation. Shaky hands, irritability, inability to concentrate – your body will make sure that you can think of nothing else until you eat and get your blood glucose level back to normal. You therefore need to be able to do two things:

i To recognise when you are in a state of low blood glucose (you are probably experiencing this at the moment at about 11am and 4pm most days, so this shouldn't be difficult);

AND

ii To have a means of getting your blood glucose level back to normal.

Remember that incredible statistic – you need 4–5.5g of glucose in your bloodstream at any one time. That's one *teaspoon* of sugar. So have something to hand that will take you back into the normal range, but without going out of the top of the normal range and therefore requiring insulin to be released and sending you into a high/low blood glucose cycle. A small raw carrot would be one option. My personal favourite is a square of 85% cocoa content dark chocolate. In this strength of chocolate, 100g has 19g of carbohydrate. If you can tolerate even stronger dark chocolate, 100g of 90% cocoa content chocolate has just 14g of carbohydrate. This means that one square of the 85% chocolate has less than 2g of carbohydrate. That's going to be perfect for taking you into the normal blood glucose range when you're a bit low, but without taking you out of the top of the normal range.

Even in Phase 2, you may like to keep some dark chocolate to hand, so that you can survive a long work day and/or avoid having to succumb to lunch meeting sandwiches because you'd be too shaky to eat nothing. If you can't have dark chocolate near you because you'd eat too much, get a bar of 100% cocoa content dark chocolate for these emergencies. If you could eat that for pleasure in any quantity I'd be amazed. It won't be pleasant, but it will do the trick and get you back to even blood glucose levels.

With stable blood glucose levels, you will be able to skip a meal quite safely and happily. You may well eat more at the next meal as you will naturally be a bit hungrier, but you won't have eaten sandwiches with 50 different ingredients or plane food, which you just didn't need. Skipping a meal the smart way is going to feel good – you'll reconnect with hunger briefly (no bad thing) and you'll feel very proud of yourself for not eating the rubbish that colleagues or fellow travellers eat.

10 Stress

The final area key to understanding why someone may not be losing weight is again hormonal. Stress is a significant health issue in today's world. Email was supposed to make our lives easier, but it has come to dominate them and to enable lots of things to be put into an inbox of things that we have to deal with, without us being able to stop it. In my first job after graduation, if I left the office to do some research (because there was no internet), no one could contact me. I could spend a happy day in a London library doing research for a business presentation for my slave-driving management consultancy employer and return and be judged on my findings alone. No phones, no emails, no BlackBerries, no iPads – just peace to do some quality work.

Life today is frantic and we have far too many 'messages' coming in virtually nonstop. The radio is telling us things, the newspaper, the TV, the phone rings, the PC pings to say 'you have mail', the list of things to do each day never goes away and we have a constant feeling of too much to do and not enough time.

What's this got to do with hormones, you may be wondering, and the answer is cortisol. Cortisol is a steroid hormone produced by the adrenal gland. Cortisol is also called a glucocorticoid, which is interesting when we break this word down into parts. The name comes from a combination of abbreviations of *gluco*se, adrenal *cort*ex (the outer layer of the adrenal gland) and ster*oid*s. We are familiar enough with the words 'glucose' and 'steroids' to know they are not good news for weight. Sure enough, glucocorticoids play a key role in glucose metabolism and thus fat storage and utilisation.

Cortisol is released in response to stress, and to a low level of glucocorticoids in the bloodstream. Its primary functions are to make blood glucose available, suppress the immune system, and aid in fat, protein and carbohydrate metabolism.

Cortisol and adrenalin are the hormones released by the adrenal gland in response to the fright/fight/flight response. Cortisol has some useful benefits therefore – it gives a quick burst of energy, it gives a burst of increased immunity, it gives a short term lower sensitivity to pain and it helps to maintain homeostasis (the body's maintenance of a constant internal environment within the body). All good stuff, if faced with a wild animal to fight or run away from.

Cortisol changes naturally throughout the day – it is normally present in higher levels in the morning and at its lowest at night. When cortisol is artificially elevated at other times of the day (in response to stress), it is important that the body's functions are able to return to normal following a stressful event. Unfortunately in our modern world, we have so many things that can stress us during the day that the body doesn't always have the chance to restore karma in between crises. Someone carves us up on the road, someone pushes in front in a queue, we have an automated voice system giving us 15 different numbers to press when we just want to speak to a human being, the delivery doesn't arrive on time – and that's just the little things. Workload may be unbearable, a child may be being bullied, a family member may be ill – that's the big stuff on top.

What's this got to do with weight, you're now wondering, and here's the answer: higher and more prolonged levels of cortisol in the bloodstream, as occurs with chronic stress or repeated stress responses, not only impact weight, they impact abdominal fat in particular.

Cortisol concentrations in body tissue are controlled by a specific enzyme that converts inactive cortisone (another glucocorticoid produced by the adrenal gland) to active cortisol.[7] This particular enzyme is located in human fat tissue, otherwise known as adipose tissue. It has been shown that visceral fat cells (visceral fat is also known as 'trunk' fat – the fat around the tummy and torso) have more of these enzymes than fat cells located elsewhere. Hence, higher levels of these enzymes in the fat cells around the abdomen may lead to obesity in this area as greater amounts of cortisol are produced at the tissue level. Adding to this, abdominal fat has been shown to have four times more cortisol receptors than subcutaneous fat (fat under the skin) – another reason why cortisol is bad news for waistlines.[8]

There is an additional reason as to why cortisol is one of the key determinants of fat generally, not just abdominal fat. It is the Hypoglycaemia connection. We know how Hypoglycaemia causes food cravings – blood glucose levels drop, driving us to raise blood glucose levels by eating any carbohydrate. Imagine that you are in a stressful job or you are more susceptible than the average person to the everyday stresses in life – you will be in a continual state of stimulus and then dip, another stimulus, another dip. During the 'dip' phases, your blood glucose levels will be genuinely low and you will be craving food – carbohydrate essentially. It is no coincidence that your first thought after a difficult meeting or phone call or event is to want to munch something. This is why people suffering from shock are given a cup of sweetened tea.

Dr Malcolm Kendrick puts stress top of the list of causes of heart disease.[9] Hence, stress is not just something unpleasant, which may stop you losing weight or cause weight gain. Stress is a killer. If your job is killing you, you need to rethink what you do. We all start from the point that we couldn't possibly change jobs and yet, most of us will have faced redundancy or a job loss at some point in our lives and we survived. We likely had to cut back on expenditure, we likely had to make some tough decisions, but we got through it. Sometimes redundancy is the best thing that can happen to us because it forces the decision on us that we should have made anyway, but for fear. In the extreme cases of work-related stress, some of you may need to think about what you do for your health, not just your weight.

This will only be in exceptional cases and the rest of us can still do much to manage stress. One of the best tips I was ever given was to turn off every incoming message that you don't need to receive. Don't have the radio on in the background, not even in the car. Don't turn the TV on unless there is a programme that you really want to watch. Turn off the phone if your job/life allows it and let an answer machine take messages and then return calls when it is convenient for you. Switch off email when you are working on something and then nothing pops up to distract you and you will be more productive. If you can't get some 'me-time' every day, at least have more days in the week when you do something that you really enjoy than days when it all seems like hard work. Your weight and life will benefit.

The last resort diet

One of the things I am most often asked when seeking advice for plateaus is 'what should I eat to maximise my chances of losing?'

The first resort is always: go back to Phase 1, dropping the NLY if you have been craving/eating tubs of it and keeping the 'no mixing' rule from Phase 2. Most people do report a loss within a few days of going back to a strict Phase 1. Keep a very accurate food diary during this time to be absolutely sure that there are no slips that have crept in to your daily eating pattern.

The last resort diet is as follows: if at least a fortnight of strict Phase 1 has made no difference (and there is *no* short-term reason for this, eg warm weather or the time of the month), then start the 'last resort'. This is The Harcombe Diet with approximately 20g of carbohydrate per day, which is approximately a mug of green vegetables/salad at each of two main meals and no other carbohydrate. This is the Atkins' strictest level of carbohydrate, so it has been well researched, back to the Banting work of the 1860s through to Pennington's work in the 1950s as being the ideal minimal level of carbohydrate. This should force even the most carb sensitive/insulin resistant person into fat burning mode.

If the last resort doesn't work, there is something else going on, as covered in the points 1–10, and probably more than one of them. Work through each of these carefully to see what it could be and don't succumb to giving up and eating rubbish out of disappointment. It's completely understandable, but it won't help and you know that.

PHASE 3

KEEPING THE WEIGHT OFF LONG TERM

WHY EATING LESS
DOESN'T WORK

We want to be slim more than we want anything else in the world and yet two-thirds of us are overweight. This doesn't make sense. We want to be slim so badly that we will replace food altogether with fake shakes or eat nothing but cabbage soup for a week or even surgically alter our stomachs so that we can no longer digest food properly. Our desire to be slim knows no bounds, but our efforts are going unrewarded. In fact, we're getting fatter. The more we try to slim, the fatter we're getting.

In 1972, 2.7% of British men and women were obese. By 1999, those figures had increased to 22.6% for men and 25.8% for women.[10] That's almost a tenfold increase in obesity for women in less than thirty years. During that time, we have barely stopped dieting.

So we have two paradoxes:

1 We want to be slim and yet we're not

AND

2 The more we try to be slim, the fatter we get

Could these be connected? Yes they could and we have known this for almost 100 years. Francis Benedict was believed to be the first person to document the impact of a calorie controlled diet.[11] He put 12 young men on diets of approximately 1400–2100 calories a day with the goal of lowering their body weight by 10% in one month. Their diets were then adjusted to maintain the lower weight for another two months. As soon as the men were released from the experiment, they overate and regained all the weight lost in less than two weeks. Within another three weeks, they had gained, on average, eight pounds more than their starting weight. At the end of their imposed diet, the energy requirement of the men had dropped so dramatically that, if they consumed more than 2100 calories a day (a third less than they had been eating), they put on weight.

This was thought to be the *first* experiment of its kind. The Minnesota Starvation Experiment was the *definitive* study of calorie controlled dieting.[12] Ancel Keys selected 36 conscientious objectors – men aged 20–33 who didn't want to go to war – to take part in his experiment on the campus of the University of Minnesota. The experiment lasted for one year. The men lost weight initially, though nowhere near as much as the calorie formula promises will be lost. Within weeks, many were having to have calories reduced further and further to try to induce any more weight loss. Some men started to gain weight on as few as 1000 calories a day. When the men were released from the experiment, after 24 weeks, and allowed to eat freely again, they binged uncontrollably and regained all the weight lost, plus approximately 10% more.

Does any of this sound familiar? Have you failed to lose 2lb (1kg) a week, week in, week out, without fail no matter what your gender, age, starting weight or any other detail? When you start a calorie controlled diet, do you become obsessed with food and notice that the next meal time can't come soon enough? Have you ever got to the point that you seem to have to eat less and less, not to lose any more weight, but just to try to maintain your weight – or avoid weight gain? Have you ever dieted, lost weight and regained it and more? Gone on another diet, lost weight, regained it and more?

That's what happens and we have known that this is what

happens since 1917. We also have almost 1,000 pages of academic documentation of the ultimate diet, The Minnesota Starvation Experiment, published in *The Biology of Human Starvation* in 1950 to prove, beyond doubt, that eating less does not work. Eating less will lead to us weighing more.

As an obesity researcher and an author of diet books, I spend a lot of time talking to people about their weight problems. The most common thing I am ever told is, 'I didn't really have a weight problem. I thought I needed to lose a bit of weight so I went on a diet, lost some weight, but then regained it and a bit more. Then I went on another diet, lost some weight, but then regained it and a bit more . . .'

This is how the so-called developed world has become fatter and fatter despite wanting to become slimmer and slimmer. To break out of this cycle, we must stop what we have come to know as dieting – cutting calories/trying to eat less. We have to do something different. And you're doing the right thing – you're reading this book.

The vast majority of diets are calorie deficit diets – they are trying to get you to eat less (and/or do more) because they think that the body will just magically give up body fat because you want this to happen. The body won't, as the two experiments above have shown. The body will do whatever it takes to make you eat. This alone will ruin most dieting attempts. If you manage to overcome your hunger and misery for long enough to lose some weight, your body will be adjusting to the lower fuel input with you powerless to stop this. This is why you get to the point that you put on weight on a calorie intake that used to lose you weight. This is why your friends and family cannot understand how you eat so little and yet still can't lose weight. The body doesn't have to give up fat. The body's job description is to keep you alive and giving up fat is seriously bad news in the attempt to keep you alive. So your body is fighting you all the way.

I bet, if you add up all the pounds that you've ever lost, it will equal your entire body weight a few times over. Phase 3 is arguably, therefore, the most important phase of the three. This time you are going to maintain your weight loss.

Phase 3 came from sanity. The definition of madness is doing the same thing and expecting a different result. We have known since Benedict's first experiment in 1917, through The Minnesota Starvation experiment, to evidence collated in recent obesity journals, that trying to eat less is *not* sustainable and does *not* lead to sustained weight loss. You will only know one, maybe two people, who have lost a lot of weight with calorie deficit dieting and kept that weight off. The rare person who has managed this will likely be hungry, miserable and obsessed with food for the rest of their life. They will have to continue to eat far less than they actually need just to maintain any weight loss, let alone to lose any more.

Knowing this from research and knowing this from experience leads to the obvious conclusion that eating less is not the way to achieve long-term weight loss. Eating better is the only way.

The huge advantage that you have as you reach Phase 3 is that you have *not* eaten less along the way. You have therefore *not* slowed your metabolism any more than your lower weight will lower your energy need naturally. You have *not* used up lean tissue while starving, which would further lower your metabolism. You have *not* had your body working against you to keep you alive. On the contrary, your body is thrilled with the abundance of real food that it's getting and the absence of junk food.

There is, therefore, no inevitable regain, as happens with any calorie counter who reaches target weight and then can't starve any longer. Every time I see a success story in the media, where someone has reached target weight and is raving about how wonderful they feel, I feel so sorry for the person, as I know that they have approximately a one in fifty chance of keeping off any substantial loss.[13] We all think that we can be that rare person who does maintain their weight loss. I thought the same when I reached my lowest weight. But, as Ancel Keys found, you have to eat less and less to avoid regain, let alone to lose more, and the human body will just not allow us to do this. It will fight us all the way.

Calorie counters can arrive at their weight maintenance phase undernourished, tired, prone to illness and with all three conditions that we write about in this book.

The calorie counter therefore arrives at their equivalent of Phase 3 – time to maintain weight – with insatiable food cravings. Try as this dieter might, the cravings are going to be quite overwhelming. The person absolutely determined to stay slim is now a food addict, with virtually no chance of resisting the many drivers to eat.

You may well be familiar with this situation – you lost weight, were determined to keep it off, and then biscuits, crisps and/or chocolate were 'talking to you' and you just couldn't silence them. You gave in – just today, only today – determined that you would be back on track tomorrow. However, giving in to the biscuits, crisps and/or chocolate nicely fed Candida, nicely embedded Food Intolerance and nicely continued your Hypoglycaemia. You woke up the next day just as likely to crave and binge on processed carbohydrates as the day before. And the day after. And so on.

It is not your fault that you were possibly able to lose weight, but not keep it off. Now you know – counting calories turned you into a food addict. You won't have done this by the time you next get to maintain weight loss: and so welcome to Phase 3.

EVERYTHING YOU NEED TO KNOW ABOUT PHASE 3

Phase 3 has just three rules:

1 Don't cheat too much

2 Don't cheat too often

3 Be alert and stay in control

Phase 2 forms the basis of your eating for life, so you carry the Phase 2 rules through to Phase 3 with you. Your basic way of eating should be to eat real food, avoid mixing fats and carbs and avoid the foods that are problems for you. Cheating is eating anything that breaks these Phase 2 rules. Phase 3 is all about becoming an expert at cheating, so that you can feel the freedom and liberation that this brings, but always staying in control. Feeling out of control around food is anything but liberating, so we will avoid getting back to this state at all costs.

1 Don't cheat too much

Rule 1 is about how much you cheat. Eat a biscuit if you want one, but don't eat ten. Enjoy a nice meal out, but don't have a dessert if you're already uncomfortably full. You no longer have 'good' days and 'bad' days, so there is no longer a rationale for having days when you don't eat much and days when you eat everything in sight. That's not being nice to yourself at all and we're grown-up dieters now – we nourish ourselves, not punish ourselves.

If you're going to cheat, you don't need your normal meal as well. That would be cheating too much. When I'm in London, there is a French-style patisserie near one of my regular meeting places. I won't have lunch that day – I'll have an all-butter croissant with a milky cappuccino instead. It feels so luxurious and indulgent. I've mixed fats and carbs, I've had some white flour, but I've also had butter and milk and some good nutrients. So I haven't done any harm and it just feels so amazing that I can have a croissant and love it and not eat so many that I feel sick. Those Cambridge Fitzbillies days are long gone.

When I worked at the Welsh Development Agency in the noughties, our office was in the centre of Cardiff and, on a particularly stressful day, I would get a small box (100–150g) of Belgian cream and cocoa-rich chocolates and have the whole box for my lunch. There is no point whatsoever having a salad at lunchtime as well – so have a significant cheat instead of a meal – not as well as. Was a box of chocolates a good lunch? In terms of nutrients, of course it wasn't, but it was pretty marvellous for my mind health on those days I can say.

2 Don't cheat too often

This brings us to rule number 2: don't cheat too often. This is about how frequently we cheat. There is no way that I would have a croissant, or a box of chocolates, for lunch every day, or even a few times a month. Cheats should be rare and even more enjoyable for their scarcity. If you have the same cheat too often, it will become habit and you will be amazed at how quickly you can develop a taste for sugary, processed food again. It creeps up on you far quicker than you would realise.

Not all cheats are equal and you will be able to get away with some more frequently than others. The more processed the food, the less you should risk cheating with it. So red wine (grapes and not much else) or very high cocoa content chocolate (cocoa, cocoa butter, sugar and vanilla) are closer to real food than chocolates or cakes. (The main ingredient in chocolates is usually sugar and there will be many other ingredients that you are better off avoiding.)

My favourite cheat is 85% cocoa content dark chocolate and I have quite a lot almost every day. My husband's favourite cheat is red wine and he has quite a lot of that, almost every day. You will learn through trial and error what you are able to get away with, but the closer to real food you cheat with, the more likely you are to be able to make this an integral and regular part of your Phase 3.

The other cheat that you will be able to adopt more regularly is mixing. When I reached Phase 3, as a vegetarian at the time, I couldn't wait to get back to crispy baked potatoes and melted Cheddar cheese for warming winter lunches. When we get back hungry from a day out, there is nothing simpler than grabbing a packet of oat biscuits (ingredients oats, vegetable oil and salt) and slapping some cheese on top with a few grapes. Both are examples of mixing and both are less risky than a processed food item cheat.

Sometimes you may want to enjoy cheats when you want them. Other times, your lifestyle will make it convenient for you to have cheats when they arise naturally. For example, someone may be celebrating a birthday at work and you may want to feel the same as everyone else for the first time in your life – enjoying a slice of cake, knowing that it won't send you out of control and it won't make you gain weight.

I had the privilege of being on the board of governors at Cardiff Metropolitan University from 2006 to 2012. With this honour came more black tie events than one had posh dresses for and sumptuous meals at each one. I loved being able to eat these three- to eleven-course meals using my Phase 3 expertise. I would never eat the bread rolls – who needs these when so much tasty, real food is on the way? I would leave any pasta, rice or potatoes – why fill up on starch when you can leave room for dessert? I would essentially have a fat meal – any meat, fish, eggs, cheese, vegetables or salads on offer – and then enjoy the dessert if I liked it. Any cream dessert I would enjoy, eg chocolate mousse, tiramisu, ice cream, etc. Any pastry/flour dessert I would pass on – I've never been a fan of stodgy puddings. Use your cheating wisely and don't waste it on anything that you're not that bothered about.

Phase 3 will thus enable you to feel like a 'normal' person – if there is such a thing when it comes to food. You will be able to have a slice of celebration cake on your terms. You will be able to go to events involving food without any of the fear that used to accompany such things. You will be able to cheat – just not too often.

3 Be alert and stay in control

The final rule in Phase 3 is to be alert and stay in control. This means that even when you do cheat – not too much and not too often – you must still stay hyper alert to your relationship with food. The minute that you sense that you are starting to need something regularly, rather than desire it occasionally, act immediately. Cut this food out straight away and don't reintroduce it again for days, if not weeks (the longer you leave it, the safer it will be).

You will need to be really honest with yourself to become adept with rule 3. As you start to develop a liking for something, the temptation will be very strong to kid yourself that you're not developing a mild addiction again and you'll want to tell yourself that it's fine to continue having the food. Let's say you've had problems with dairy foods in the past. You may reach Phase 3 and pick up a cappuccino on the way to work and relish the sweet taste of milk sugar, which you can taste when free of the many sugars in processed food. This may start as a rare treat and then it becomes more regular. It won't take long to get to the point that you pick up a milky coffee routinely each day. You may then even find yourself having another cappuccino later on in the day. You are possibly at stage two of addiction by now – you want something and you start to want more of that something. You must stop now before you reach stage three and start to feel bad when you don't have the milky coffee. Indeed, you may stop the coffee the next day and feel low – a sign that you were already entering stage three of addiction.

If in doubt – cut it out. Don't allow any food to control you again. You are going to be the one in control of food for the rest of your life.

What to cheat with

For every food that you would like to be able to consume again, there is a processed version and a less processed version. Cheating needs to be based on the closest thing to real food that you can find. This is not only for weight reasons, but for health reasons. As an example, you can get crisps/potato chips with just two ingredients: potatoes and sunflower oil (they don't even need added salt). Or, you can get crisps/potato chips with this list of ingredients: Dehydrated Potatoes; Vegetable Oil; Rice Flour; Wheat Starch; Barbecue Flavour (Sugar, Flavourings, Smoke Flavouring, Spices, Wheat Flour, Dextrose, Flavour Enhancers: Monosodium Glutamate, Disodium Guanylate and Disodium Inosinate, Citric Acid, Malic Acid, Colour: Paprika Extract, Acidity Regulator: Sodium Diacetate, Onion Powder, Tomato Powder, Paprika Powder, Mustard Seeds, Barley Malt Flour, Yeast Extract, Celery); Emulsifier: E471; Maltodextrin; Salt; Modified Rice Starch.[14]

Please don't ever be that horrible to yourself. Do you even know what those ingredients are? Let alone if they are good for you or not?

You can get quality ice cream with these ingredients: cream; skimmed milk; sugar; egg yolk and natural vanilla. Or you can get cheap ice cream with about 50 different ingredients, many of which you can't pronounce or explain.

If you have bread, get some Irish wheaten loaf from a bakery or farm shop. This will be closer to old-fashioned wheat than the modern processed bread in supermarkets. Better still, make your own bread, maybe even with rice flour and seeds to avoid wheat.

Become a dark chocolate connoisseur, enjoy wine with evening meals again, savour berries and fresh cream for dessert. Buy the best food that you can afford and dine at the best restaurants within your budget. No Michelin-star restaurant ever serves processed food. Real ingredients, put together with love and skill, will be the best things you ever taste. You'll know that you will never be a junk food addict again when your idea of heaven is a rich, creamy, salmon mousse on a bed of peppery leaves.

PHASE 3 PERSONAL EXPERIENCES

My experience with Phase 3

Phase 3 shocked me. I had been such a junk food addict that I thought it would be idyllic to get back to the things that I used to crave, but this time to have them on my terms and not to feel controlled by them. It took me several months to break my sugar addiction, so I spent a long time on Phase 2 even after I had reached my natural weight. I started to enjoy mixing before I went near processed food and this was when I first discovered dark chocolate. I had found it too bitter previously – a comment many dark chocolate virgins make – but persevere and you will never go back to cheap confectionery again.

I knew that my sugar addiction was over when my blood glucose levels were wonderfully stable all day long – I no longer experienced any symptoms of Hypoglycaemia or manic sugar highs. I also had the most amazing constant energy all throughout the day. I would wake up raring to go and feel the same way up until bed time. The energy, and even mood, that I felt post food addiction was just priceless. I was pretty confident at this point that I could try some things that I had enjoyed previously and be fine with them. I *was* fine with them. The shock was that I no longer enjoyed them. I used to love boxes of chocolates – Quality Street, Roses, Celebrations were the main UK brands. I tried some and they tasted sickly sweet, synthetic and nothing like I remembered.

Having got rid of my unnaturally sweet tooth, I had come to appreciate nature's natural sweetness: cherry tomatoes; milk sugar – lactose; berries in season; even beetroot and parsnip chips taste sweet in the real food world.

Harcombe fans' experiences with Phase 3

'AAARGH! Phase 3!! It's what you dream about when you first embark on The Harcombe Diet and when you get there, the feeling is so good I wish I could bottle it! Shopping trips where you keep seeing yourself as fat and then the realisation when you are looking in the three-way mirror and cannot comprehend your new slim body!! Compliments, new clothes and great health. What more could you ask for?? And then it all just falls apart again. In the euphoria you feel invincible. You dabble in a bit of this and a bit of that, and still don't gain weight. You become used to getting away with it, until you've overdone it and the weight piles on. What are you armed with on Phase 3? Three rules only and those three rules seem like nothing at the time, but those three rules are everything. Ignore them at your peril. I did and the weight piled on. What happens then? Well you have to start again, but at least now you know WHAT to do. Knowledge is power and that's what The Harcombe Diet provides for you, the knowledge to manage your eating for the rest of your life. This is the miracle of Phase 3.' *Lizzi*

'Phase 3 for me has been just a natural extension of Phase 2. There is really so much choice of delicious food that I really haven't seen the need to regularly cheat!

'There have been a few times when I have been out for a meal and thought – sod it! I'll have the chips with the meal! I have done this and not put weight on. This is because I'm not doing it too much or too often!' *Mat*

'I cheated too much and too often when I first reached Phase 3 and regained some of the weight I had lost. I have since learnt that I can still get away with a lot as long as I don't do it every day and at every meal! I can have dark chocolate every day, the occasional dessert and a few glasses of wine every now and then. If I ever put on a pound or two, I just do Phase 1 for a few days until they are gone again! My body no longer tolerates rubbish and I definitely feel the difference if I have eaten processed food.' *Sian*

PHASE 3 TIPS FROM OUR HARCOMBE FANS

'Don't ignore the rules, unless you want to put more weight on! Enjoy yourself, but use all the knowledge you've gained on Phase 2 about what foods work for you and what don't. Compromises may have to be made, but they are worth it. It's easy to go out and let yourself go, but be prepared to do a long Phase 1 at the end of it. When in doubt, it's always better to cheat on real food than rubbish. Your body will thank you for it!' *Lizzi*

'This is a tip for when you are out and about. I don't always feel that hungry at lunchtime and, if I'm out, I always carry a couple of squares of 85% chocolate to have with my coffee/tea. It's more than enough to get me to my evening meal. I find that most coffee shops only sell carbohydrate-laden food – a real problem when eating The Harcombe Diet way.' *Jane*

'Start gently – a Phase 2+ – introduce new foods gradually and monitor the effect.' *Howie*

'My tip would be that when cheating, if possible go for lower carb cheats such as wine, dark chocolate and nuts. All of these are low in carbs and unlikely to make you gain weight in moderate quantities. Desserts, cakes, biscuits, milk/white chocolate, however, are another matter and are to be approached with extreme caution! Watch out for cravings returning and nip them in the bud as quickly as possible with a day or two of Phase 1 or 2 (whichever works best for you; personally I find Phase 1 the best for getting rid of cravings).' *Sian*

'If you cheat on processed food, remember how it makes you feel. Most of my cheats these days are on real food purely because it doesn't make me feel bad afterwards!' *Alix*

'Don't be afraid to try things that you used to have a problem with. I lost my intolerance to some dairy by the time I got to Phase 3.

'Phase 3 for me is really a state of mind – my young son would probably call it The Harcombe Diet Ninja level – expertly educated!! If you get into trouble with food/weight you know how to fix it.' *Helen*

'Don't think of it as your diet having ended – it's the way of the rest of your life beginning.' *Mamie*

PHASE 3 QUESTIONS

Q What is my natural weight?

A Your natural weight is the weight that you can maintain fairly easily. You go above it if you indulge – maybe on holiday or over festive periods. You go below it at times of extreme stress or illness. You can cheat, but not too much and not too often, and still find it relatively easy to maintain a natural weight.

If you find that you continually have to cut things out, or repeat Phase 1 on occasions, to try to maintain your current weight, it is less likely to be your natural weight. If you have spent most of your adult life at a particular weight, going below this may be unnatural for your body. I do believe that the natural weight range for the majority of people will be in the normal or overweight BMI category – obese BMI levels are less likely to be natural. Remember, males and taller people tend to have naturally higher BMI levels than females and shorter people.

Natural weight can change over time. We often recall nostalgically our weight at our eighteenth or twenty-first birthday party, or at our first prom/college ball, or on our wedding day. The chances are that we did a daft calorie restricted diet before some of these events and our weight on these days may not be a good indication of our likely natural weight. Women are likely to change shape and weight, to a smaller or greater extent, following childbirth. Illness or injury can also impact one's natural weight over time.

Q How much can I get away with?

A This is completely individual. The experiences and tips from Harcombe followers will be helpful in showing you different results for different people. I can get away with quite a lot – I eat dairy products and dark chocolate daily. I mostly avoid wheat, but can get away with it on occasions. I can enjoy other grains – rice and oats – quite freely. I have many meals out and eat what's on offer. My husband, Andy, doesn't eat grains. However he can enjoy beer on rugby match days (beer is grain based) and get away with it. He drinks wine most days and has a lot of cheese. The low carb blogger, Jimmy Moore, can get away with virtually no carb intake before he starts to fight weight regain. Some people in the club have ended up more at the meat/fish/eggs/veg end of the spectrum and some are enjoying bread, cereal and lots of carb meals, not least our many successful vegetarians.

It really will be a case of you working out what you personally can get away with and weighing up the pros and cons. It may be that you can maintain a weight slightly higher than you would like, but enjoy quite a lot of variety and freedom in your diet. To maintain a lower weight might require sacrifices that you're just not prepared to make.

Q How do I know if I'm craving something or just fancy it?

A Be honest. If you really feel like you could take or leave something, then leave it just to be sure. If the thought of leaving it gives rise to a low level of panic, you are starting to need that substance, rather than just want it.

Needing things, as opposed to merely wanting them, can creep up on you far quicker than you might expect. I blogged once about receiving an enormous (1.5kg) box of quality chocolates one Christmas and enjoying a couple here and a couple there. It was barely a few days before I started to fancy a couple with morning coffee and then another couple after lunch and I was heading rapidly back to sugar addiction.

Nip even the slightest concern in the bud immediately – the longer you leave it, the more likely it is that 'take it or leave it' can turn into 'need it' and you'll be fighting cravings again. The key to Phase 3 is to never let those cravings return.

OPTIMISING SUCCESS

HOW TO STAY ON TRACK

Starting a diet is easy. I've lost count of the number of diets I've started in my life. Staying on a healthy eating plan is the first difficult thing and developing lifelong sustainable principles to maintain weight loss is the other challenge. Phase 3 gives you these lifelong principles to keep the weight off. This chapter is all about keeping you on track, whichever phase of the diet you are in.

WHAT MAKES US FALL OFF THE WAGON?

There are many and varied things that trigger 'falling off the wagon'. You know what I'm talking about – you're doing really well, you're determined and focused and then something happens and you're off track before you can work out what went wrong. This chapter is to highlight these obstacles on the track, which can so easily derail you, so that you can be acutely aware of them and have strategies to counter them.

There are a number of things that trigger falling off the wagon and we'll go through the main ones to make sure that you don't succumb to these dangers:

Christmas
These tips can help with any festive occasion during the year, when the killer combinations of family and food come together.

The biggest risk generally is that the festive period throws you off course and it takes weeks, or even months, to get back on track. The biggest risk specifically is that food addiction can return even in a very short period of time. The risk is greater for our North American friends, who start celebrations early with Thanksgiving (the last Thursday in November). A very useful study appeared in *The New England Journal of Medicine* entitled 'A Prospective Study of Holiday Weight Gain' (March 2000). This article quantified that the average weight gain for Americans can be 5–7lb (2–3kg) over the holiday period. Given that many people don't gain weight, some people could be gaining their share and someone else's in a couple of months.

It can be astonishingly quick for food addiction to take hold again. The longer it has been since you were addicted to food, the safer you will be. The better your immune system, the less likely it is that addiction will happen. The less you have been cheating, the more you may be able to get away with a few days of processed food without becoming addicted again (you will most likely feel 'rubbish', however). If you have been bingeing more recently, are a bit run down at the end of the year and find it difficult to resist things here and there already, you are at the highest risk of Christmas being quite a damaging time for you.

Candida can definitely overgrow again in a few days. You may be surprised at how quickly Food Intolerance can redevelop – have a mince pie for more than a few days in a row and you are highly likely to want another one the next day. Symptoms of Hypoglycaemia can literally occur in an hour or two. If you have had nice, stable blood glucose levels for a period of time and then eat some confectionery, you could have a big high followed by a big low within a 30–90-minute period.

If the conditions are allowed to take hold again, you will reach the end of the festive period with more than a few presents to show for the holidays. Yes, gaining a few pounds is a risk and would be unwelcome, but I would worry even more that you regain food addiction and gain even more weight before you manage to get the cravings back under control again. It's just not worth it. So, let's look into this further . . .

You should have one of two goals over the festive period to maintain your weight or to continue losing weight. Gaining weight should not be in your consideration set.

1 Maintaining weight should be no problem. If you are at your natural weight, and have some Phase 3 experience, use all the tips that you have picked up to manage your cheating to the best of your ability. If you are not at your natural weight, but want to relax slightly over the festive period and are happy to maintain weight before going back to losing again, check out the Phase 3 guidelines and make sure that these are at the forefront of your mind. You've got the three rules: don't cheat too much; don't cheat too often; be alert and stay in control. Here are a further three top tips for Christmas:

- Don't have the same things every day. Almost all processed foods contain sugar and white flour, so these are the high risk ingredients for you to regain a taste for. However, if you're going to cheat a bit, don't have a mince pie or Christmas cake every day, try to vary things so that you don't form a habit for something in a short time. Cheat with mixing (turkey and roast potatoes) more than with processed food wherever possible and then you won't suffer the carb bloating and hangovers that will be likely.
- Don't allow bad days to develop. A cheat doesn't make a bad day. A cheat is a conscious decision, which is absolutely fine for you to make. If you want some chocolates, have some, but have them as your meal, not as well as your meal, and don't pick at them one at a time all day long, drip feeding blood glucose problems for the whole day. Your other meals for that day should be normal meals. So you might have porridge for

breakfast on Christmas morning and then you may opt
for the turkey dinner with roast potatoes, stuffing and
chipolatas. You may even have a bit of pudding. But then
stop eating after lunch and dinner/tea should be cold
turkey and salad, or something else that meets Phase 2
rules, and you're not then cheating all day long.

- My overall top tip for cheating, after 15 or so years in
Phase 3, is just because you can cheat, doesn't mean you
have to. Cheats are often disappointing after eating so
well for so long. Great cheats are nut roast, milky
porridge with tasty mixed seeds, crispy baked potatoes
with grated cheese. My favourite cheats are mixed
versions of real food. I really have no interest in a white
flour, sugar-laden mince pie whatsoever. I just don't think
that anything is worth the impact on my blood glucose
levels and how high and then low I would feel. Find your
equivalent of dark chocolate and red wine, so that you've
got a cheat that feels special to you.

2 Losing weight is actually remarkably easy over a festive
period. Most celebrations that we have are based on
feasts, but those feasts tend to be meat based, as this
would have been the most luxurious food possible
throughout history. Both Thanksgiving and Christmas
celebrations feature roast turkey dinners with all the
trimmings. You can lose weight happily by avoiding the
trimmings.

Losing weight over the festive period is all about
choice. You can see the period as a long haul from the
first party through to New Year, when you vow to go on a
diet. One day slips into another, one excuse into another:
I can't be 'good' Thursday because it's the work party. I
can't be 'good' Saturday because there's a dinner. There's
no point getting back on track for one day on Friday and

so on. That kind of thinking is sure to make the festive a long period during which you feel progressively worse and gain progressively more weight. Doing Phase 1 for even one or two days during a festive period will keep you wonderfully on track.

The infinitely better way to think about any festive period is that it is the same as any other time of the year. There are just a few days when one meal (it's rarely more than one meal) is slightly out of your control. Even then, meals are rarely really out of your control. The work dinner is likely to be a Christmas dinner, so you can fill up on turkey, sprouts, carrots and parsnips and leave the stodgy stuffing and roast potatoes for those who want their outfits to start feeling uncomfortable. The vegetarian option is usually a nut roast or similar. It will probably mix fats and carbs, but one meal is not the end of the world. Decline the pudding – don't even let the serving staff put one in front of you or you will feel obliged to eat it.

Your secret weapon at any meal or drinks party is communication. Ask people questions about themselves and really listen to the answers – give the person your undivided attention. Talk and share things with friends and new acquaintances. You will be remembered as the great listener and interesting guest, not as the person who didn't even notice that dessert had been cleared away while they had been so engrossed.

When you see the festive period as a few dinners and parties, rather than a full month of 'feeling out of control', it makes the whole thing seem far less daunting. You carry on with your real food eating plan, eat the real food on offer at the odd dinner that you attend, and then there is no reason why you shouldn't start January lighter than December.

Even Christmas Day is really just one meal – lunch. Breakfast should be what you normally have and then you shouldn't need anything until Christmas lunch is served. You can stick to Phase

2 rules at lunch, or have some potatoes, chipolatas and trimmings. Real food cheats are much better than any pie or cake cheats. The problem you may find on Christmas Day is that most people overeat to such an extent that they don't want a third meal. You will likely need one, so cut some cold turkey or cheese and find some salad and cherry tomatoes and have a good fat meal. People who have missed a meal are usually the ones munching on snacks all evening, while watching some rubbish telly. Make sure that you don't sit within reach of any nibbles and don't fall into the mindless eating trap.

Straight after Christmas Day comes Boxing Day and that's the time to put on your comfy trainers and enjoy a good walk around the sales. The time between Christmas and New Year is a great time to lose weight before the New Year's Eve party. Then it's January 1st and the whole thing is over for another year. So it's not really a festive period – it's a Christmas lunch and a couple of parties.

Complacency and curiosity

I have put these two words together, as I think that there are some interesting parallels. There are broader observations to be made from starting to feel complacent and/or curious at the same time.

Here's the scenario: You're doing really well. You may even be at natural weight. You don't crave things any more. You feel that you're not a food addict any more. You could take things or leave them, but instead of leaving them, you take them. I first thought of this as complacency – we relax into thinking we aren't addicted to food any more, so we can't become addicted again, so we become complacent and try a few things. Then, before we know where we are, we have developed a taste for our former demons. For some people it may be just that one drink or just that one cigarette and they feel hooked again.

It may be curiosity driving this. We know what sweet stuff

tastes like – we used to binge on it. We almost test ourselves – I wonder what would happen if I had toast for breakfast. I'm in a coffee shop – why don't I have a muffin? The trouble is, you only need to do that a couple of times before you associate being in a coffee shop with having a muffin and you find yourself going to a coffee shop to have a muffin.

The curiosity is fuelled by so many different things:

- 'I used to like milk chocolate, I haven't had milk chocolate for a long time – I wonder what it tastes like.' This is a natural human emotion, but it needs to be nipped in the bud with a quick reminder of why you gave up confectionery. It's processed junk; it is bad for your health and weight; you don't want to reward food manufacturers for their bad behaviour; it's addictive; it gives you all sorts of other unwelcome symptoms and so on.
- 'It's normal to eat cereal. Lots of people have packaged cereal for breakfast and a cereal bar mid-morning – why can't I?' Advertisers spend millions to make sure that you think this. Coffee shop staff ask you at the till if you want anything else because they know that 7 out of 10 snack purchases are made on impulse. Every time you go into a petrol/gas station or a newspaper/magazine shop/outlet, you will likely be asked, 'Do you want a bar of chocolate with that?' or whatever special offer piece of junk they are trying to offload that day. The sales representatives for crisps and sweets will have told the garage staff that most snacks are not planned purchases, so they should tempt people into making one.
- 'It's healthy.' This is one that I personally struggled with – what could be healthier than a bran muffin? Surely I can have a bran muffin as a snack? – until you learn that you no more need the bran than you do the mass of white flour, sugar and salt disguising the taste of the

'inedible' bran bit. Watch adverts and see the emotions that advertisers are trying to implant in your mind as connected to their product. Coca-Cola is life; a Mars a day (that one got challenged); cream cakes are naughty but nice; beer drinkers have a great sense of humour; spirit drinkers are sexy and impossibly glamorous; eat Special K and you'll be wearing red and swimming all the time. Try telling yourself the opposite message at the time of watching the advert – a Mars a day *won't* help you work, rest and play; 'winos' on a park bench drink spirits; and so on. Funnily enough, it then doesn't quite have the same appeal.

You can't ever afford to become complacent. You were an addict, you could be an addict again. You don't want to develop a taste for junk again, so what's the point in trying it.

You can't afford to be curious either. There are only two things that can happen:

i You try something, feel awful and the only benefit is the reminder that this stuff is bad for you – you knew that already.

ii (Worse) you try something and like it – this means that you're not over the addiction yet and you still have a taste for it and you will want more.

If you really are curious, do what some bloggers do, using themselves as experimental guinea pigs and sharing the results. They try raw liver; they stop hair washing to see if it really does end up not needing to be washed (the answer is yes); they eat only things with faces for a couple of weeks; they try going without dairy to see if it makes a difference. If your curiosity only tends to manifest itself in trying things that you tried lots when you were a food addict, this should tell you something.

Events/special occasions

This seems to be an issue more for people in the early stages of The Harcombe Diet. It doesn't seem to take regulars long before they become a dab hand at events. Most people come to realise that many events are actually easier for those watching carbohydrate intake than those watching calories.

Special occasions can include weddings, dinner parties and work dinners. Those are the common challenges, so let's get some coping strategies:

WEDDINGS You've got the killer outfit for your friend's wedding and the last thing that you want is for the seams to be straining after the first course. Here are some top tips to avoid the bloat in your skintight outfit:

- Have the good meal

  Weddings usually consist of two meals: a sit-down dinner after the ceremony and a buffet later on. You don't need both. The sit-down meal is generally real food-based and healthy. It may be smoked salmon starter, chicken or lamb main course, then dessert (berries and cream ideally). Just avoid the bread, potatoes and heavy puddings and you'll feel no strain on your outfit. The couple will have chosen the meal weeks in advance, so ask what it is if you want to plan ahead.

- Don't have the bad meal

  Wedding meals are usually late and then, before you know it, there's a buffet appearing with sandwiches, sausage rolls, vol-au-vents, cakes, crisps and more white flour than you will be able to remember seeing for some time. Don't even approach the table – no one will notice that you've not gone up for yet more food. You're far better off being too busy dancing or chatting. Have a small bar of 85%

cocoa content dark chocolate in your handbag – a couple of squares will give you a healthy lift if you're flagging.

- Avoid the canapés

  Sometimes food comes round with the Champagne even before the meal. If you see anyone carrying a canapé, turn away. You can clock up 50–75 calories every time you chomp one. That's not the problem – it's the fact that they're 'useless' calories – things in batter, breadcrumbs or on toast. If it's a sensible budget wedding, and no sit-down meal is planned, have a light cheese/chicken/tuna salad before you arrive and you'll have less urge to munch during the rest of the day.

DINNER PARTIES Dinner parties are fine if you're the host. If you're not, then if you know the hosts well enough (as hopefully you will), tell them what you are doing and say that you would love any meat, fish, eggs, cheese, vegetables, salad on offer, but will be passing on the carbs (you may need to explain that these are the bread, potatoes, rice, pasta and so on). Ask if you can bring anything to help.

If you don't know the hosts well enough to be honest, the easiest way to avoid carbs is to say that you are wheat intolerant (you almost certainly are). This cuts out bread, pastry, pies, cakes, biscuits – the most important things to avoid. You may still be offered potatoes and/or rice and you will likely be able to have a bit of either for one meal with little problem. If you don't want to eat these either, decline them if possible when being served, or leave them.

I can't stress enough that a good host is one that puts the feelings of their guests above their own. A good host should want the guest to be as comfortable and as 'at home' as possible. A good host should not mind if food is eaten or left, not be offended if something is tried or not tried. A good host would not try to force an alcoholic to have a drink and they should not try to force a food addict to go back to things to which they are addicted. A good host is *not* the home equivalent of the 'office feeder'.

WORK DINNERS Work dinners should be even easier than private dinner parties. At best, they will be held in restaurants where plenty of fat meal options will be available and you can choose something ideal. At worst, they will be a set meal in a hotel or similar venue. You may get the chance to choose in advance or the meal will be a 'safe' one suitable for many different dietary requirements. Chicken and salmon have been the two most common offerings at the vast number of dinners I have attended (for most of these I was vegetarian and the vegetarian option was usually some kind of pastry, tart, pasta or risotto – all far more fattening than the meat/fish meal). At work events, there is no one to offend. The wonderful waiting staff clear the table to set times, so make sure that you're talking too much and your meal is 'unfortunately' cleared away before you can eat anything that you don't want to. As mentioned in the Christmas section, that really is the top 'meal' tip – talk and listen. You can't eat at the same time.

Even if you find yourself eating something that you normally wouldn't, the key thing is what you do next. It's just one meal – get straight back on track. Don't let the taste for sweet or floury stuff take hold again. Hopefully it made you feel a bit bad and it ends up being a really useful experience as it strengthens your resolve not to do it again.

Please don't ever decline an event because you're worried about food. I turned down so many events – even weekends at the beach with friends – because I felt fat and/or was worried that I wouldn't be able to control the food there. I don't regret many things in life, but I do regret things I said no to when yes would have been much more fun.

Habits

I have had porridge every day for breakfast for years. I like it. I don't think about it. It's fuel. Eggs would be healthier and a 'perfect' three meal plan every day would be an egg-based meal, a fish-based meal and a meat-based meal, to get all the different nutrients that we need from food. But I am in the habit of eating porridge. As it causes me no harm, it's not a problem habit.

Spend one day noticing how much you do out of sheer habit – get up, put your slippers on, go downstairs, put the kettle on, make breakfast, shower, get dressed. Driving the car is pure habit – you probably wouldn't even know what you had just done if someone stopped you and asked. Habit is vital – we couldn't function if we had to make a decision about everything all the time. Habits are really important for children to make sure that they are not overloaded with decisions and choices. This is why we don't give them the option, such as do you want to put your shoes on when you go outside. They learn really early on that going outside means putting shoes on. That's another decision that they then don't need to make.

What are your food habits, however? Can you go into a café without wanting a cake or muffin? Can you watch TV without snacking? Can you go to the cinema without buying a bucket of popcorn? Are you the person who can munch their way mindlessly through a lot of fake food during a film? You've gone to watch a film. If you want to eat, go out for dinner. I'm being harsh to make the point about how easily we connect one activity with another and adverts are always there to help us. You're at the cinema and the first five minutes of adverts are telling you to eat ice cream, M&Ms, get a drink – food manufacturers want every activity that we do to be firmly connected with eating and drinking. Go bowling – have a drink and a snack; go shopping – stop for a coffee. They know that habits formed are difficult to break. We need to break them and ideally not let our children develop them in the first place.

Every time I went swimming as a child we were allowed something from the vending machine afterwards. Boy did that take years to break. Swimming and a bag of crisps went hand in hand in my mind for a long time.

To break a bad habit, you first have to recognise that you have one. Think of every activity that you do – socialising, cinema, TV, going here, going there – and make a note of every food or drink that you connect with that activity. Know what your habits and associations are.

The next step is to then break those habits and associations. There are two ways of doing this. Either:

i Continue with the event, but be aware of the habit and don't follow it (eg go swimming, but don't have the crisps).

OR

ii Stop the event for approximately 21 days so that the pattern can more easily be broken. My mother only gave up smoking when she stopped going to the teachers' staff room because that was where she most smoked. If you can't watch TV without snacking (and you've tried knitting, surfing on the PC, cat on the lap – all the other suggestions), then stop watching TV.

Holidays

For many people, holidays are a time when they gain weight. Some people gain at each holiday, then struggle to lose the weight before the next holiday and it has a cumulative effect. I must admit I struggle a bit to understand holiday weight gain. I lose weight most holidays because there are usually no Harcombe-friendly carbs, so I have more fat meals. I also eat far less dark chocolate on holidays – if skiing, the chocolate gets too cold and on beach holidays, it melts. Not good for either. Andy and I also tend to take full-board holidays (to give him a well-deserved break from cooking), so we have the natural pattern of three large meals a day.

I can sort of understand gaining weight on skiing/cold weather holidays. That's when carbs can be quite tempting as they warm you up and provide instant fuel for exercise. I can't understand gaining weight on a beach holiday. Surely that's when you feel most self-conscious and most want to look your best – on the beach and dressing up in the evening? That's when the warming effect of carbs is most uncomfortable. That's when the water retention and bloating caused by carbs is just horrible.

I know people who go on holiday *planning* to come back a few pounds heavier. There seem to be a few interesting thought processes going on here:

- 'I'll let go on holiday and then lose it when I get back.' If this is your thought process and you have been on enough holidays by now to know that you do lose any gained weight within one, maximum two, weeks of being back and you think the 'gain' at the time is worth the 'pain' when you get back, then make this conscious decision and do it. It wouldn't be my decision, but positive choices are much better than things feeling out of our control. If you don't always lose any weight gained, and find yourself with your weight creeping up every time you go on holiday, you need to decide *not* to choose this option again.

- 'I'll never have this opportunity again.' One of the things that most panics humans is the sense of scarcity. There's worry about petrol, so we all rush out and buy some. Food is running low before Christmas, so we make the situation worse by buying more than we need. When humans think things are running out, they hoard. There is something akin to this on holidays. There is a special meal served one evening and we think we will never see it again. If it's a hog roast or a seafood buffet – great. Eat as much as you like, skip all carbs and you'll be fine. If it's an example of all the finest desserts that the pastry chef has managed to come up with, here are some tips – have it instead of your meal, not as well as; just because you can, doesn't mean you have to; don't eat to the point of feeling ill – that's not fun.

The scarcity worry is that we have this sense that we will never in our lives see food like this again. If this is really the case, then you may *choose* to make the most of it. Our honeymoon coincided with an epicurean buffet with the world's best chefs staying at our resort in Jamaica and cooking banquets every night. We both ate some of the best food we have ever tasted and I was glad that we got married on day 3 of the holiday or I wouldn't have got into my dress on day 10! That really was a one-off. We choose our holiday locations for the food. We go to places where we know the food will be great, but that doesn't mean that we have to eat any more or any differently to how we do at home. It's just more real food. Good hotels don't do junk.

- 'I've paid for this, so I'm having it.' The final thought process is about waste. If we have gone for bed and breakfast, half-board or full-board, we think we need to get value for money. 'I've paid for three courses, so I'm going to have three courses.' You've also paid for the pool, the exercise room, the babysitting service, the concierge – do you feel you need to get the most out of all of those? Probably not – food has a unique connection when it comes to waste. If served a meal, eat what you normally would and leave the rest. If the meal is buffet style, only take what you know you will eat. Go back again if you need to, then you will have nothing to waste. The only person impacted by food going in your tummy or staying on the buffet table where it is, is you. Don't eat anything just because it's there. Of all the bad reasons for falling off the wagon, that's a top one.

If you have made a decision that you are going to eat what you want on holiday, then at least mug up on Phase 3 and minimise the damage. If you don't want to gain weight on holiday, here are the tips:

- You won't find good carbs, so stick to fat meals – you may even lose weight doing this.
- Stick to the three meals a day. You should find this easy as you'll either be on the hotel meal plan or you'll be eating in cafés and restaurants at the resort. If self catering – even easier – stick to local meat, fish, eggs, salads and things you would have at home.
- Know that the minute you eat white flour/pasta/ processed carbs, you will gain a few pounds with the (heat-related) water retention, so it's just not worth it.
- Wear close-fitting clothes, or a belt, eating out and then you can't overeat or eat the wrong things.
- Choose the venue with the food in mind. Real food is difficult to find at a Disney resort – Epcot being an exception. If you don't fancy burgers and fries for a week, you may want to avoid Disney World. If you're a vegetarian, don't go to Russia (also personal experience).

Illness

Illness is one of the most genuine and challenging reasons for falling off the wagon. A number of things can happen:

- You feel so ill that you will do anything/eat anything to feel as OK as you can
- Your health, quite understandably, becomes more important than losing weight
- You may be given medication that makes the weight problem worse
- You feel low, so you feel that you need cheering up more than usual

The single biggest tip here is that, with The Harcombe Diet, gaining health and losing weight go hand in hand. This is not an either/or, to put your effort into, it is the means to the end. The more you eat real food, the less you eat processed food, the better you will feel whatever the illness – from flu to cancer to diabetes. Illness may make you feel less inclined to 'diet', but don't see it as a diet. See eating great food as the way to nourish yourself back to health and not as something you're doing to lose weight. One will follow the other.

If you read up on illnesses, almost all advice given for getting better will include dietary advice. Most will say eat well, eat real food, eat fresh food and so on. I've not seen any that say eat biscuits and cakes and crisps and see if getting stodge inside you will make you feel better.

I would highly recommend reading about vitamins and minerals if you are suffering more than a very short-term illness (such as a cold or flu). When you realise what vitamin A is needed for, or calcium, or manganese, you will be stunned and shocked to wonder why no one has made sure that you get enough of all of these in your diet every single day. Put energy and effort into optimal health and nourishment – not recommended dietary allowances.

I recommend trying to view a period of illness as a good time to lose weight. You may well be off work, so you don't have to worry about Candida die-off impacting your performance for a few days. You have fewer expectations on you at this time, so you may be able to invest some time in yourself, eating well and getting back to health. You may go out less, so this may help to avoid the temptations of snacks to buy everywhere. You may need to sleep more and you can't eat when you're sleeping. The only good thing about flu or tummy bugs is that we lose a few pounds and, when we recover, we remember how great it is to feel well. If you are ill for a while – wouldn't it be wonderful to recover from the illness and be a few pounds down when you do? There is no reason why this can't happen.

The 'sod-it' mentality

This is such a tough one. When we are losing well on a diet, it spurs us on and makes all the effort worthwhile. When we stop losing, and plateau for a while, the mentality can change to 'sod it – I'm putting in all this effort and not losing, what's the point, I may as well eat what I want.' The cruel bit is – eating what we want will make us gain weight, not even maintain weight. Every time we plateau we are at the mentally tough place where we get no 'reward' for our efforts and yet, if we stop those efforts, we get 'punished'. You know how it goes. I used to suffer from this badly myself.

The 'sod it' mentality achieves nothing and makes things very much worse. I've been there. I would be disappointed with the result getting on the scales one morning and I would feel a wave of relief as I 'allowed' myself to eat whatever I wanted that day. I would usually go out to get a croissant and/or pastry (more likely a few) and start my 'fun' day straight away. There would be no proper meals throughout such a day. There would just be continual eating – one minute feeling so sick I didn't think I could eat any more and less than an hour later feeling compelled to get something else sweet (when the blood glucose dip kicked in). I would get through crisps, boxes of cheap chocolates, ice cream gateaux, bread – all sorts of horrors. It would cost me a fortune; I would lose the entire day (it's a full time job having a binge) and I hated every minute of it. Actually the only 'fun' bit was that sense of relief once I'd given myself the day off. This is the moment to stop the binge before it starts. Know that you can have that sense of relief – you are a grown-up now – you can eat what you want, whenever you want. However, *then* decide not to make the bad choice and you will feel infinitely better by *not* going ahead with a binge.

You have every right to feel the 'sod it' mentality. It makes complete sense. But you have to choose *not* to go down that route and here are three reasons why:

i You will gain weight. 'Sod it' is not something you can do for even one day, let alone a few days, and not suffer serious consequences. Disappointed as you are that the scales are not showing a loss, how much more upset would you be if they showed a gain? And show a gain they will. You could easily gain as much as five or six pounds in one day and you then have even more to lose than you had before the binge.

ii You will feel terrible. Having been off processed food for a period of time, going back to it may feel enjoyable for the first mouthful (maybe not even then – usually the relief is really truly the only OK feeling). The actual food consumption usually starts feeling terrible as soon as it starts. You hate yourself, you become a food-stuffing zombie, you feel sick, you bloat – it really is anything but fun.

iii You will reawaken cravings. If you have avoided processed food for several weeks, even months, you will probably get away with a slip day slightly more easily than someone who slips after just a few days or weeks. The sooner you slip, the more likely you are to be still addicted to certain foods and still have the conditions to overcome and therefore the more likely that a slip is going to have consequences.

To get the taste for flour and sugar soon after having given it up is too risky. The body is highly likely to continue to want more of this stuff. So, you may have your 'sod it' day and the body thinks 'Great, we're back to the processed stuff that gives me sugar highs and feeds my Candida parasite' and the body doesn't want to turn back.

Please have these thoughts in your head while you are thinking clearly and that is when you are eating real food and not in a carb stupor. Before you get on the scales, you have to vow to yourself that there is nothing that can show as a reading that will impact your resolve. If you doubt yourself, don't get on the scales.

The more that you can think of weight loss as 'chipping away', the less likely it will be that not losing makes you think 'sod it' and makes you fall off the wagon. Weight loss, achieved through eating real food and managing carbohydrate intake, stays off. Just keep losing a bit and then expect a plateau, lose more, likely another plateau. Just keep chipping away downwards knowing that, this time, there is no reason for lost weight to go back on – not if you stick with real food/managed carb for health and weight. Enjoy the reassurance of knowing that what you lose need not go back on, unlike those who go back to processed food or do low calorie dieting.

You can also try a careful Phase 3 if a plateau turns out to be quite a long one. Give yourself a break and try to maintain with more flexibility and being less strict for a while. If you can still maintain in this situation it can have two benefits:

i It takes the pressure off you for a while

AND

ii You may well get a good kick start when you go back to the more rigid plan of Phase 1 or 2

Sugar pushers/Office feeders

I get annoyed by a few things in the world of dieting, but it's more a 'how can people be so ignorant' kind of irritation, rather than a real annoyance. For example, when people say 'overweight people just need to eat less/do more', I pity the naivety of the person trotting out this pointless platitude, rather than feel angry.

One thing that does get me quite angry, however, is people pushing processed, sugary, floury foods on other people. Can you imagine the reaction if they were trying to encourage an alcoholic just to have one drink? 'Go on, try it; just one drink won't hurt; I made the punch specially – just have a little...' You'd have their doctor to answer to. Yet we have at least 10 times as many overweight people as alcoholics and people think that it's OK to fuel the obesity epidemic in this way.

To help understand where the other person is coming from we need to remember that food in our society is seen as nurturing and social. We feed children and our loved ones and we offer food to visitors and so on. Rejecting food can therefore be seen as rejecting a nurturing offer. Knowing this can help you to soften the blow: 'It's so kind of you to offer, but I've just had lunch/I'm just about to have tea', etc. Redirect the nurturing offer. Instead of accepting a biscuit, let the nurturer know, 'I could murder a cup of tea – thank you so much.'

With parents, the nurturing has a stronger connection because parents feel responsible for feeding you – they did for 16 to 18 years, why stop now? The line between nurturing and control with parents, however, all too often gets blurred.

They probably decided when you ate, as well as what you ate and how much you ate. Your strong views about food now can be seen as a kick back against that control and against them knowing what's best for you. I genuinely do believe that, a few monsters aside, parents do want to do the best for their children and anything they 'get wrong' is with the best of intentions. If your parents have been trying to get the non-evidence-based five-a-day into you and feeding you starchy pasta for tea and cereal for breakfast and you turn around and ask for bacon and eggs and pork crackling, they are going to take this personally. It is as if you are criticising their parenting and their healthy eating beliefs and you are. There's no getting around this. You will likely find yourself wanting to help them – to tell them the truth about five-a-day and fat. Much as you want to share the news, when you realise the lies that we have been fed, I would caution against you trying to convert family or long-standing friends. If they show interest, that's one thing, but you trying to encourage others to put butter on vegetables is no different to them trying to encourage you to eat potatoes. Try not to make food the battleground that it may well have been for much of your life.

Here are some tips to help you counter the sugar pushers/office feeders, however and wherever these well-meaning people seem determined to make you fall off the wagon:

- A well-known British retailer, selling books, cards, stationery and confectionery, has a nasty habit of putting enormous blocks of chocolate at the till. The staff have obviously been instructed by Head Office to ask if you want a colossal bar of sugar, no matter what you put on the counter to purchase. My husband, Andy, has a great response when he is asked to buy such rubbish. He tells the assistant, 'I didn't get a body like this by eating junk like that!' If you're still work in progress, you can opt for a variation of this, 'I got a body like this by eating junk like that!' If someone has made the item (for example a cake at work), you can remove any offence by saying 'irresistible stuff like that'.

- The simple words 'No thank you' can be repeated indefinitely until the sugar pusher gives up. 'Would you like some cake?' 'No thank you.' 'Oh, go on.' 'No thank you.' 'Just a slice.' 'No thank you.' 'I made it myself.' 'No thank you.' Keep smiling sweetly. Any more than five requirements to say 'No thank you' and I would be tempted to say, 'Which bit of no thank you did you not understand?'

- Gluten intolerance is an increasingly common issue, so saying that you are gluten intolerant can be really helpful (you almost certainly are wheat intolerant). It cuts out anything with flour, so that you can decline bread, cakes, biscuits, pies, pastries and so on and there's nothing that the sugar pusher can do.

- Humour can be quite disarming, even though this isn't a laughing matter. 'Gosh – don't let me near that cake if you want anyone else to have some.'

- Devious compliance is good at larger gatherings. If you can't be bothered to fight, take your plate of whatever is being pushed, walk away and leave it on a windowsill or sideboard somewhere. Some binger (or dog) will find it!

- Another option is to have an adult conversation. This is especially useful with family occasions where you know that the pressure is going to arise. You can even have the talk in advance to avoid difficult moments. 'Mum, I love seeing you at Christmas and you know I'm trying to do something about my health and weight and I could really do with your support. I'd be so grateful if you didn't offer me any sweet stuff…'

- As a last resort, I actually think that you have every right to be very direct. Imagine that you are an ex-smoker and someone is trying to push a cigarette on you. Imagine that you are an alcoholic and someone is trying to make you drink. Share those examples with the sugar pusher. 'If I were an alcoholic, you wouldn't dream of trying to get me to drink. Food has been my addiction in just the same way, so please don't try to push food on me.'

The Time of the Month (TOTM)

This is not just for the females in the club – every male who knows a female encounters premenstrual tension (PMT), also known as premenstrual syndrome (PMS).

Some women barely notice the TOTM, but I don't know many women who fall into this category. For many the TOTM blights their life. The few days before a period are dominated by PMT/PMS – physical symptoms such as water retention, weight gain, bloating, sore breasts, swollen thighs, clumsiness (banging into things) and emotional symptoms such as depression, feeling blue, weepiness, feeling overwhelmed, feeling less productive and less able to cope generally.

Do an internet search for 'menstrual cycle hormones' and you should find a picture of what is happening to different hormones in the female 28-day cycle. Prepare to be amazed by how much progesterone, oestrogen, follicle stimulating hormone (FSH) and luteinizing hormone (LH) change in a 28-day period (the cycle length can vary for different women). Both the absolute level of hormones, and whether they are rising or falling, impacts on physical and emotional symptoms. A woman's gender hormones can change more each month than a man's in a lifetime, so we should not underestimate the impact of this cycle on females.

Of all the things that make us fall off the wagon, this is the one that we need a plan of action for. It happens for up to one week in four, every month. That's not like a wedding or a Christmas party – that's a way more frequent 'derailer' of dieting good intentions.

If you know what your symptoms are and when they occur, write them down so that you know what you're up against. If not, keep a diary for at least three months and then the pattern will be clear. Note physical and emotional symptoms, cravings, weight changes – anything relevant.

When you know your most difficult days personally, develop coping strategies for those days especially. For example, work may not always allow this, but try to schedule the things that demand most effort and productivity on the 25–26 days when you don't feel overwhelmed and weepy. Can you schedule admin/clearing emails on your least productive days? I feel quite overwhelmed and useless for a couple of days each month, so I've stopped fighting it. I know that just a couple of days later I will be ready to take on the world again – and so will you.

Don't worry about losing weight in the few days around the TOTM. Take that pressure off yourself. Use the Phase 3 principles to manage cheating and to maintain weight during this time. What you don't want is to gain a couple of pounds each time, which keeps disturbing your ongoing weight loss. Find cheats that work for you – more dark chocolate is one good option and with the iron, zinc, manganese and magnesium it contains, it's likely what your body is crying out for anyway. You may want porridge breakfasts for a couple of days at this time. Even if you find yourself eating more than you 'should', make sure that the things you go for are still 'good' options.

Oat cakes, larger main meals, snacks when you feel you need them – try to listen to your body and work with it. Processed food, especially carbohydrates, will honestly make you feel horribly worse and really must be avoided at all costs. Do whatever it takes to make sure that you don't succumb to these.

In summary, know that these couple of days happen and give yourself a break in terms of workload and food. You *know* that the only way to stop the cravings for rubbish is to *not* eat the rubbish in the first place. There's no other option. Know that the days are going to pass and make them as bearable, if not enjoyable, as you can. If you see a friend once a month – arrange it at this time; if you go to the movies once a month – go when you're feeling low. Make these days to look forward to, not days to dread.

Treats

A common reason for falling off the wagon is that we have an association, which has been built up over a long period of time, such as that we see sweets as treats in a strongly connected way. We're having a tough day, we could do with cheering up and we suddenly fancy a biscuit. We've been running errands all over the place, we see a coffee shop and we tell ourselves that we deserve a coffee and cake. There are two powerful ways of dealing with this:

i First, we need to find non food/drink things as treats. I wish parents would start this from a very young age. When a child falls over it wants a cuddle and sympathy. The child is upset, so food is actually the last thing on their mind, but we give them a sweet to cheer them up – not least because that's what our parents did.

   We each need a list of things that are treats for us – none of which involve falling off the wagon. Put a coin in a piggy bank every time you get really close to having a biscuit, or other junk, and get a massage when you've saved enough. Take time to watch your favourite programme, even when you know that there are chores to do. Go and have a chat with someone in the office who always cheers you up. Promise yourself a glass of wine if you don't give in to something worse. The treats can still be food/drink, but they need to be closer to healthy eating than junk.

ii See the junk for what it is – it is the opposite of a treat. It might feel nice for about 30 seconds (if you're lucky) and then it feels dreadful and you regret it. That isn't being nice to yourself. That is being horrible to yourself.

There is a well-known saying – a moment on the lips, a lifetime on the hips. If you can think really consciously about this phrase, it is powerful. When something tempts you, consciously work out how long it would take you to eat it. A minute? A couple of minutes? Then think about how easily cravings could return, how your blood glucose level could start going all over the place, how your energy for the day could be affected and ask yourself – is the 20 seconds that it would take to eat a couple of chocolates worth it? The answer has to be no, so leave them. It really does take seconds to eat things that can then spoil our resolve – it really, really is not worth it.

The final tip on this one is to promise yourself that you will delay giving in to something. In the café, promise that you'll get your coffee and then only go back for the muffin if you really, really want it and have decided that it is worth it. My bet is you won't even queue up for it again – that's how easily the moment can pass.

The Bottom Line when it comes to wagons and falling

Despite all these practical tips, for many different scenarios, if you do fall off the wagon, the two most important things to remember are:

i Never miss an opportunity to learn. Every time that you fall off the wagon, learn from it. Write it down to embed the learning more firmly – why did you fall off? What was the trigger? How can you avoid the trigger? If you can't avoid the trigger, how can you avoid it having the same effect next time that you encounter it? Do you remember the moment when you knew that you were going to fall off the wagon? What could you do next time, at that point, to stop it?

ii Remember – no one ever ruined a diet with that first slip. It's what you (yes *you*) decided to do next that ruined the diet. A moment of falling off the wagon is not an open invitation to eat anything or everything that you used to eat, but haven't eaten for some time. There is no benefit at all in regaining the taste for processed food. Chances are the slip was understandable – you were caught out and about and all you could get was a sandwich. Having the sandwich doesn't mean having crisps, confectionery and anything else that perhaps you used to eat with a sandwich. Having a piece of cake, to share in a celebration, is not an excuse for getting a packet of biscuits or box of chocolates on the way home and eating the whole lot. One thing does not ruin anything – unless you decide to make it so – so don't do it.

FINALE

THIS COULD BE YOU

Let's pull everything together and get you ready to embark on the last diet that you'll ever need . . .

You now know that eating less doesn't work – it never has, it never will. It makes you want to eat more and this alone will ruin most diets. It would have ruined The Minnesota Starvation Experiment had the men not been locked on a university campus and unable to access the food that they so badly desired.

Eating less also drives behaviours, which cause the three conditions that turn you into a food addict. Not eating enough weakens your immune system, making Candida overgrowth more likely. The carbohydrates that the dieter chooses also feed Candida nicely. Getting the biggest bang for the buck, the most food for the fewest calories, makes the dieter choose the same foods every day. As too much of the same foods are eaten too often, so Food Intolerance develops. The carbohydrates favoured by the slimmer – fruit, rice cakes, cereal bars, sweets, etc – are also the foods that play havoc with blood glucose levels and lead to Hypoglycaemia. That's why calorie controlled dieting hasn't worked for you so far and it never will.

You now know all this, so you will not try to eat less again. You will now eat better. You won't count calories, but you'll make those calories count. Eating real food to nourish your body will help you to lose weight and gain health.

You will attack these three conditions and keep them at bay with our 3-step plan:

THE HARCOMBE DIET 3-STEP PLAN

1 Phase 1 – staying on this for at least five days – longer if you have more than 20lb (9kg) to lose and/or you have moderate or severe Candida overgrowth.

2 Phase 2 – staying on this for as long as you need to, to reach your natural weight. Adopting the three powerful rules of Phase 2 until they are second nature and the foundation of the way that you will eat for the rest of your life.

3 Phase 3 – cheating not too much or too often and staying alert and in control. You never want to be a food addict again or out of control around food again and there is no reason why you should be.

You now know how to reach and maintain your natural weight and how to live craving-free for life. You've just got to follow the 3-step plan and go for it. As if the prospect of being slim and healthy for life isn't enough, we've asked our club members to share their personal stories to give you that final bit of inspiration.

As you read their warm and wonderful stories, just think – in a few weeks' or months' time, this could be you.

The Harcombe Diet saved my friend's life

'Timi, who happens to be my best friend, was diagnosed with an advanced stage of heart failure with an enlarged heart. It was clearly the result of her obesity (22 stone (140kg) and 5ft 7in at that stage) paired with a difficult physical job. I had a serious chat with her and explained that if she didn't lose weight very soon she was very likely to suffer a heart attack with an almost 50% chance of dying. At the age of 36.

'This was a real wake-up call for her. She started The Harcombe Diet on the very same day. She has tried various diets before without any success and her biggest problem was that she got stuck on a low-calorie diet – she was starving herself and still gaining weight. Once on The Harcombe Diet, she started preparing her own (full-size!) meals, she hasn't touched any processed food or sugar ever since and, 4–5 months later, she weighs 15½ stone (100kg). She knows she still has a journey ahead, but she is already immensely happy about what she has achieved.

'Timi's symptoms are mostly gone: the fatigue, shortness of breath, mobility problems, pains and constant infections. She is waiting for a cardiology checkup to see the improvement on her heart. She feels stronger and fitter than any time in the last 10 years and even more enthusiastic about The Harcombe Diet. We both honestly believe that The Harcombe Diet saved her life.' *Edit*

Farmer back to fighting weight – with asthma beaten

'I am a farmer in my mid-fifties and have gone up and down in weight all my life. At 17, I was 18 stone, but soon lost much of it when I started working on the farm. I was 12½ stone in my early twenties, but soon piled it back on. I lost a lot in my thirties, basically by eating less and doing more, but it piled back on again. November 2011 I was 16½ stone, totally unfit, and on quite serious medication for asthma. A friend of mine recommended The Harcombe Diet as she was successfully shedding a lot of weight on it. Phase 1 was pretty uneventful for me, no headaches etc, and the weight started falling off. On to Phase 2 and from November to about March 2012 I had got down to 12 stone, where I am currently 'holding'. Waist gone from 40in to 34in and I feel 10 years younger. Other benefits being that I no longer need steroids for asthma and I've not taken my puffer in months.' *Barleycorn*

The hospital plan didn't work – The Harcombe Diet does

'I have been fat in various degrees all my life from the age of five. I have done all the diets and the best one for me seemed to be Slimming World where I lost 4 stones, but it still allowed the eating of processed food, so I never really got rid of my food demons.

'In the summer of 2011 at 23 stones, I was referred to my local hospital weight loss service and joined their 24 week programme: 8 weeks x 5 pints of milk with 2 miso soups or stock cubes a day; 8 weeks of half milk and one meal of about 500 calories; 8 weeks of around 1800 calories. At the end of the 24 weeks I was turned loose having lost only just over a stone. I tried to stick with the 1800 calories, but it was a pain.

'Then I heard by accident about a talk by Zoë Harcombe. I went along and signed up then and there. What attracted me? That it is based on science, the rules are SO very clear and within the restrictions there is so much choice. I have no idea how much I have lost, but if you see a woman walking down Tottenham Court Road in London and her skirt falls round her ankles please come and say hello and join in the laughter. It will be joyous, believe me!' *Ellie*

Goodbye to seven stone!

'I was always a skinny thing and never weighed more than 7.5 to 8 stone until I hit 28 years and then everything went downhill. Over 15 years I managed to gain over 12 stone. The final straw for me was when I had pneumonia in January of 2011 and I was given steroids by the doctor. By May of that year I was finally steroid/medication free, but I had ballooned and in my eyes was the most hideous creature on the planet.

'I went for my usual hairdressing appointment and my

hairdresser showed me Zoë's book *Stop Counting Calories & Start Losing Weight*. I had nothing to lose so went and bought the book on my way home . . . what a light bulb moment.

'Two days later, and surrounded by sceptics, I started Phase 1 and lost 15lb . . . it clearly worked so onwards to Phase 2 where I have been for well over a year, happily so I may add. I have lost close to 7 stone so far and have dropped from a size 22 to a 16 in my clothes. My health has been fantastic in the last year and I've rarely been ill. I still have a fair way to go but seeing the results so far, I truly believe this is now achievable. Before The Harcombe Diet my friends and family thought there was no hope for me . . . now I smile knowingly at them. Thank you Zoë and Andy.' *Josie*

Our 'Harcombe' baby!

'My story is far more about health than weight. I always had long periods of feeling very down with low self-esteem. I also suffered with migraines and would get at least one a month.

'I knew that I had a problem with sugar because once I started, I couldn't stop, and if I overdid it, I would have hangover-like symptoms for a couple of days! Despite knowing all of this, I had never before been able to give the stuff up! After five days on Phase 1, I (almost) lost all of my sugar cravings, which was amazing! I have been following The Harcombe Diet for over a year and a half now and generally don't want sugar anymore because I know how rubbish it'll make me feel!

'My husband has been following The Harcombe Diet for almost as long as I have and earlier this year we decided to start a family. I'm sure the speed at which we got pregnant had a lot to do with the hugely healthy diet we'd both been eating for over a year and I know that once I've had the baby in February, I'll know exactly how to get rid of any excess weight.' *Alix*

I was given six months to live

'I've always had weight problems all my life and can remember my Mom getting Energen rolls to help with a diet I was on when 16 years old; I've been your typical yo-yo dieter.

'In March 2008 I went to the doctor and thought I may have diabetes. He took blood tests and blood pressure readings. When I went back he said do you want the good news or the bad? I said I'll have the good news. He said I hadn't got diabetes. The bad news was I was 19st 7lb and my blood pressure was 178 over 135. He said these were death figures and told me not to make plans for later on in the year as I wouldn't be here in six month's time. So I went home and told my wife I was going to die and started to cry. I joined a local gym, as this had helped the two times I had been in this state before, and started going every afternoon Monday to Friday for about 3½ hours. By November 2011 my weight had come down to 15 stone.

'I had stalled in my weight loss, was getting myself down and was on the verge of packing it all in as I wasn't getting anywhere.

'I came across The Harcombe Diet when my wife showed me an article in a Sunday paper magazine about Zoë's *The Obesity Epidemic* (April 2011). In November 2011 I was tidying the bedroom when I found the article again and this time tried it.

'It helped me to lose another 2½ stone by April 2012 to reach 12 stone 7 and a blood pressure reading of 128 over 57. My doctor said he had 21-year-olds on his books with figures higher than that.

'I'm no longer on a diet. It's a complete lifestyle eating

plan for me now. I've lost 7 stone in body weight and achieved a body fat percentage of 21.7%. My waist was 54in and is now about 36–37 in. So I've got to spend a fortune on new clothes soon.' *Larry*

I didn't realise that three conditions were stopping me being the slim, healthy person I should be

'I had always been slim and healthy. In my twenties I discovered I had a problem with dairy and cut it down, but not completely out of my diet. Desserts and pizzas were too good to give up completely. Ten years later I was finding it harder to keep the weight off so I started exercising more, punishing myself if I didn't go out on a run every day. I suffered increasingly with itching, sinusitis, exercise-induced anaphylaxis and IBS. I ended up taking antihistamines daily for five years and felt there was no way out. I ate less and less in a desperate bid to lose, but still the weight didn't come off.

'Three years ago a colleague came in and was half the size she used to be. She told me about The Harcombe Diet. I bought the book and my life changed. The light bulb moment came with Zoë's explanation of Candida, intolerances and Hypoglycaemia. On Phase 1 I lost half my goal weight. Within two weeks all my itching stopped. I cut out dairy and grains completely. I no longer had to take antihistamines and I could exercise without getting itchy or experiencing anaphylaxis symptoms. Within six months I was on Phase 3. In the three years since starting The Harcombe Diet I've not had any health problems, not even a cold. Not only do I look good, but I feel good too. I've got my life back!' *Lizzi*

Thank goodness I didn't qualify for bariatric surgery – even with a BMI of 48

'Towards the end of 2011 I was deeply depressed having been turned down for bariatric surgery as my BMI was 48 and had to be 50 to qualify. Putting more weight on wasn't an option – I had to lose it as my blood pressure was sky high. I looked on the internet for something I hadn't tried and stumbled upon The Harcombe Diet. I looked on the forum to get more info and ordered a copy of the book and watched Zoë on YouTube.

'I started The Harcombe Diet at the end of November 2011, weighing in at a very unhealthy 26 stone. My waist was 52in and my shirts were 5XL. I set myself a goal of losing 10 stone in 12 months as I needed something to focus on. I found the first week hard and didn't feel good for the first few days, however when I weighed in after six days on Phase 1 I had lost a stone. This was more than enough motivation for me to carry on and I didn't look back after that. I found it easy on Phase 2 and quickly found the things that were stopping me from losing weight, like shredded wheat, cheese and berries, and I cut them out. The forum is a fantastic place for support and advice and I can't imagine how it would be without that network of mates.

'After nine months on The Harcombe Diet I had lost 8 stone (now a 38in waist and XXL shirts). I am now approaching month 11 and have lost another half a stone. My loss is slowing down to a crawl now as my body approaches what I feel is my natural weight, but I intend to continue on to my anniversary and see where I am. On reflection I can't imagine being in a better place from 11 months ago, thanks of course to Zoë and The Harcombe Diet. HAPPY DAYS!' *Big Lad*

I thought gaining weight and losing health was part of getting older – it doesn't have to be!

'I started The Harcombe Diet in August 2009. I was approaching my mid-fifties and felt pretty good – apart that is, from the slowly creeping weight gain, the almost constant heartburn, aches and pains in my joints, colds and sore throats every other month, recurrent athlete's foot and, being a fashion lover, I didn't like the clothes options that were available to me. I could go on but hey, these problems are all just part of growing older aren't they?

'I'd been discussing the heartburn at a party and the person I was talking to suggested that maybe it was a wheat intolerance. The same week I came across an article by Zoë and bingo . . . something clicked in my brain. It all made such sense. I wasn't greedy. I wasn't stupid and I had been led to believe that I was living a healthy lifestyle by eating low fat and exercising like a mad woman, so why wasn't I slim and healthy.

'I sent for the *Stop Counting Calories & Start Losing Weight* book and started Phase 1 straight away. I didn't weigh myself at the outset as I long since stopped weighing as it was too depressing. I found the whole process easy to follow and it made such sense. It did take a leap of faith to believe that I could eat fat again, but I knew the low fat wasn't working for me so it was worth a go. From day one the heartburn stopped. I was only into the first week of Phase 2 and a friend asked what I was doing because she could see I'd lost some weight and she thought my skin looked good. The results were that quick to show. I was also unable to exercise at this point as I was recovering from an injury and I realised that the weight loss was happening despite my inertia.

'Eventually I went on to lose about 4½ stone in about ten months. It was a nice steady loss and I never felt like it was hard work because I loved the foods I was eating. Having to stop my reliance on processed sauces and ready meals reawakened my interest in cooking. All my problems seemed to melt away with the weight. No more aches and pains, no athlete's foot, clearer skin, shiny hair . . . every aspect of my health and wellbeing improved. I also realised that I could enjoy my exercise as and when it suited me for its own sake and not because I needed to try to use it as a method of weight control. I've found a size and shape I'm happy with and maintaining it is easy.

'I've often described the way I now feel as euphoric and that is not really too strong a word for it. I know for sure that I bless the day I read the article and set off down the Harcombe road.' *Mamie*

I learned the hard way that calorie counting is a myth

'It is two years since I discovered that losing weight is not about eating less and exercising more.

'Since then, I have come to realise that all the years of focusing on calories and filling myself with low calorie white carbs has caused me to become so fixated on sugar that I have become addicted, tired and more overweight than I was when I started trying to lose just half a stone when I was a teenager.

'My life has been dominated by weight and food issues since I was 15, and my weight has consequently increased over this time. I used to weigh 9 stone, then it was 10, down to 9 and then up to 10 and a half, then it leapt to 12, back down to 11 and there it stayed (ignoring a 13 stone smiling pregnant woman in the middle). No matter what I have done, whom I have talked to or what I have been tested for (in my more desperate moments) – it's always followed the same pattern.

'There is no evidence behind the "cut your calorie intake by 3500 per week to lose a 1lb in weight" theory. I was sold a kipper. All that happened was I became starving hungry and my body was filled up with more bowls of plain pasta, dry toast and indigestible beans.

'So, in November 2011 I was introduced to Zoë Harcombe and her thoughts on food, sugar addiction, Candida and Food Intolerances.

'My epiphany goes as follows – by going vegetarian through my sheer love and emotional attachment to animals and a fear of their death, I have essentially made myself low in magnesium and zinc as well as protein deficient. My weight has increased due to the high levels of carbohydrates and my gut flora has become abnormal so I have been suffering with a bloated tummy for as long as I can remember. Animals have still been killed and eaten regardless. I couldn't save them. I should have prioritised myself.

'As many of us know, how we feel about ourselves throughout the day often depends on how flat our tummy is when we get up in the morning. My lifestyle choice increased my weight and bloated my stomach. I started doing more and more dieting, but just ate more carbs and less fats (and as we were all told this was the way to eat I thought I was doing the right thing).

'After 25 years I became happily carnivorous.

'So, if you know any young teenage girls thinking about turning vegetarian – see if they would consider eating fish and make sure they eat lots of eggs and cheese and stay away from the processed food.' *Matisse*

The Harcombe Diet has changed my life!

'I met my now husband back in 2003, when I was 26 and a size 12. Weight started to pile on; I was up to a size 16 when we got married. We then had a beautiful little girl and I peaked at a size 20, aged 32 and over 16 stone. I managed to lose some weight, but never really felt "healthy".

'In September 2011 we had a miscarriage. I was pretty low and the weight issue was only adding to things. Over Christmas 2011 I decided that there were things in my life I could not control . . . but my weight wasn't one of them. I should be in control of my weight/health.

'I bought a celebrity diet magazine, and read an article by Zoë – that article changed my life!

'Within seven months of starting this diet, I'd reached a size 12, and felt great. I'm still a size 12 . . . and still feel great!' *Kay*

I thought I was going to be a little fat pudding for life

'May 2012, I was feeling very worried about my weight gain. I'm 50, 4ft 11in and was 10 stone 4lb and gaining. I've done every diet there is and always lost weight, but always put it on again. I was starting to feel resigned to the fact that my age was slowing down any weight loss and I was going to be a little fat pudding for the rest of my life.

'Feeling very desperate and a little scared for my health, I typed in "how to stop dieting" into the internet. Lots of info on low carb came back. I found it all a little difficult to understand, but amazingly a few days later I heard Zoë on Steve Wright. My ears pricked up and I ordered her book. Now almost five months on, I am 9 stone. I would like to lose a little more to get within my BMI, but I am thrilled as I really didn't think I would lose this much weight. I haven't been this weight for over 10 years.

'The unexpected benefits were no more heartburn, no more

gurgling tummy and no more going to bed starving, and feeling miserable and a failure, because I couldn't lose weight and keep it off. It's so liberating to know I wasn't a weak-willed glutton. It was following current healthy eating guidelines that was the problem. It's been a leap of faith, but I know I'm eating all the right things for optimum health, thanks to Zoë and others like her.

'I truly hope the word will spread to more and more people, so they can experience the wonderful feeling of freedom from fear of every mouthful you eat. I know I sound a little evangelical, but that's how I feel.'
Gettingslimmer

I've lost weight, even with PCOS

'I have been seriously overweight for 20 years. I had lots of complications following the birth of my second child and it took a long time to recover and the weight slowly crept on. Before I knew it I was 15 stone and sluggish. Then eight years ago, I was diagnosed with PCOS and advised to lose weight or end up with type 2 diabetes with all the complications that it would entail.

'I was referred to a dietician who advised a low-fat low-GI diet. I was already virtually eating this way as had always thought that it was healthy, but she advised low-fat spreads, cheese, leaner meats and more fish and more fruit than I was used to. At this point I gave up as I was already eating from a smaller plate and my food just tasted bland. What's more – I put on more weight.

'While searching for healthy eating on the internet I came across The Harcombe Diet. I started and found it really simple to follow.

'Now almost 3 stone lighter, I am delighted and am at my lowest weight for 20 years. My husband joined me and we both feel fitter and healthier and see our new way of eating as a lifestyle change for the future.' *Chickenlady*

The Harcombe Diet is the only diet that has worked

'I've been overweight for all of my adult life. I started as a size 16 when I was 18 and peaked during my pregnancy in 2000, at size 26/28 and 20 stone. I had attempted to lose weight primarily with Slimming World and had struggled to get down to around 16 stone before I stopped even trying. I started looking around and discovered the GL Diet, which was probably my first introduction to healthy fats, then I went to Atkins and Tesco GI and discovered that I actually felt healthier on those types of diets, however the weight still did not budge. I would puzzle about it constantly knowing something wasn't quite right. I eventually tried Slimming World again and Rosemary Conley and maybe saw a little movement that got me back down to 14.7, but still nothing more. What was wrong with me?? It really can't be this hard to lose weight!

'Funnily enough it was a conversation with one of the guys that shares my office that led me back to thinking more about things – he mentioned PCOS as I had a few markers and I started looking around, that led me to Candida, which eventually led me to The Harcombe Diet. Immediately things started ringing some bells – since I had gone back to Slimming World and reintroduced bread, milk and my 'syns', so many things had returned like the bad dandruff, spots, always hungry, not able to control cravings . . . it was all there in black and white. So I had to try this way of eating to see if it would help.

'One of the things that stuck in my mind was Zoë's reassurance that if you give the body the right conditions to lose weight then it will eventually do so. After the first 20

days, I started to see improved energy and sleeping, my
dandruff was improving, my hair went from greasy to dry
and my spots, although still there, were no longer so angry! I
also slowly started to lose weight. I eventually broke into the
13 stone bracket and wept on the scales, then wept on the
phone to mum, then wept as I posted on the forums!
Something so small seemed so life-changing for me as I had
accepted I was going to be in the 14 stone bracket and size
16/18 for life!' *Nicola*

I'm no longer out of control around food

'There is nothing very dramatic about my "history" and I
didn't need to lose huge amounts of weight. But, like many
women, I found that over the years my weight was steadily
creeping up. Friends and family would never call me
overweight or big, but though I was well clued in on "healthy
eating" and could walk the walk, and talk the talk, giving in
to my "need" for carbs always took over. But, there was
always one diet or another to inspire me to shed a few
pounds . . . WW, SW, The Duvet Diet, The Lunchbox Diet,
The F-Plan . . . all I had to do was pluck any book off the
shelves in any bookstore – they were there in abundance.

'I couldn't eat one slice of "healthy wholemeal" – I had to
eat five. I couldn't have a normal portion of rice – it was
literally a whole pot full, with some veg and cheese added in.
Same with pasta. Considering just how much I could pack in,
I should have been the size of a house. I used sweet treats as
"rewards" – eat something "good" (oh those "healthy carbs"!)
– have something naughty.

'In my meanderings through bookstores, looking for the
elusive 'perfect diet', I'd come across *Stop Counting Calories
& Start Losing Weight*. It intrigued me, and I went back
several times over the months and kept having a look at it.

'I realised I'd found my holy grail . . . this worked! It was easy because for once I was not hungry.

'I've been maintaining for almost 18 months now and there is no sign of the out-of-control eating habits I used to be a victim of. What more could I ask for. Oh, and there is also the new sense of confidence around food . . . it no longer controls me and I enjoy it more.' *Virginia*

I nearly died

'I started Harcombe at a crisis time in my life, after a serious illness had very nearly cost me my life. I was at an all time low and my ballooning weight felt like the final straw. In fact my GP had referred me for counselling as my depression and comfort eating were out of control.

'I was always overweight and a member of a 'big' family – grandparents, aunts and cousins as well as my dad and brother all morbidly obese. A history of failed diets started with Slender aged just 10 years old. You name it, I have done it: Cambridge, Cabbage Soup, WeightWatchers, Slimming World, GI Diet, F-Plan, calorie controlled, Grapefruit and Egg diet not to mention Reductil and Xenical. Yes, I could lose weight and pretty quickly, but keeping it off was another story. Each diet led to a loss followed by a more substantial gain.

'So it's fairly easy to deduce that I was pretty unhealthy and very unfit. Around 10 years ago I was diagnosed with M.E. (*myalgic encephalomyelitis*) and became pretty poorly. I did eventually recover and when I had a relapse in 2006 thought it was back, but tests showed I had an underactive thyroid and I was put on thyroxine for the rest of my life.

'Rather than seeing an improvement in my health, I was deteriorating. By 2009 I had developed severe migraines and frequent dental abscesses, I was referred to a neurologist who said I had trigeminal neuralgia caused by a deep tissue infection and I was prescribed beta-blockers, which I would also need to take for life. Between August 2009 and January 2011, I had over 20 courses of antibiotics for various respiratory infections and abscesses, culminating in my hospitalisation in Dec 2010 with swine flu and double pneumonia and I nearly died on New Year's Eve 2010.

'When I came out of hospital after 10 days in intensive care on intravenous antibiotics, I had an out of control addiction to carbs and sugary things. I ate cakes, sweets, biscuits and syrupy drinks and was consuming a litre of orange juice a day, for the vitamin C I thought. The more I had the more I wanted. By March I had gained 2 stone and was feeling dreadful. As an already obese person this was something I didn't need. With my reduced lung capacity, I was becoming an invalid.

'Then I discovered The Harcombe Diet through a friend on Facebook, I will always thank her for introducing me to a life-saver. I read the book and lots rang true – the cravings and the three conditions, which it seemed I might have. I was also attracted to the prospect of eating real food since I have never really liked low-fat alternatives or sugar-free artificially sweetened products.

'I lost 9lb in Phase 1, going on to lose a further 5lb in my first week of Phase 2. Losing a stone in just under two weeks was an amazing boost, but what I hadn't accounted for was the unbelievable feeling of control I suddenly had – no cravings, in fact almost an indifference to food, which was totally alien to me.

'I went on to lose 4 stone in six short months. I feel amazing and everyone comments on the way my skin glows and my hair shines. More importantly, I have completely come off prescription medications apart from my thyroxine. The migraines are gone, the depression is gone and the acid reflux is gone. I hope one day to discover my underactive thyroid is functioning normally.

'I still have lots of weight to lose (around another 6 stone) to put me in the healthy BMI bracket, but the great thing is I am no longer a yo-yo dieter; I have managed to keep the weight off.

'I can't imagine living any other way anymore.' *Cazbah*

I've recovered from 48 years of dieting!

'My story is not about weight loss. It is about recovering from 48 years of dieting! I was 66 years old when I started The Harcombe Diet in January 2011 and had tried every diet under the sun, but always came back to 11 stone and the odd pound. Losing and regaining! No fun at all and totally hung up about it.

'Since then I have evolved a way of eating that suits me and my body, and although I have actually put on a few pounds, I am totally happy with this way of eating. My daughter started eating this way in March this year, not to lose weight but to get her bloated tummy sorted. Without even doing Phase 1, she has lost a stone. Her figure is now perfect.

'I have come off antidepressants, statins and tranquillisers. I am now training to be a life coach specialising in weight control. All this because I changed my lifestyle to the Harcombe way of eating!' *Harmonious*

The Harcombe Diet has helped me in sickness and in health

'I found The Harcombe Diet after failing to lose weight at a gym and only gaining muscle. I was so fed up at flogging myself to bits and counting calories for no obvious gain. The idea of eating just real food and not counting calories attracted me very much. Being the cynical type, I was not convinced I'd lose weight, but realised that The Harcombe Diet could do no harm at all and was worth a try.

'I read the book three times, stuck to the simple rules and lost around 20kg in about nine months. I ended up lighter than when I got married 20 years previously! Equally as important as the weight loss, my health and state of mind improved dramatically, most of which I put down to controlling my blood glucose levels by dumping wheat and sugar. No more eczema or migraines, much better skin and a much more balanced mood, which the whole family appreciates!

'The Harcombe Diet has also taught me that we all need to educate ourselves about food. Many family members have since joined me in The Harcombe Diet and are enjoying the benefits. Since losing the weight that I wanted to, I have had to face a cancer diagnosis and subsequent treatment, close family illness, depression and bereavement. Throughout this difficult time, my life has been made immeasurably better by knowing and feeling that I am properly nourished, and that if I slip up with food, I can get back on the straight and narrow and I will feel better.

'The Harcombe Diet is not a fad, or even a diet. It's a way to live under any and all circumstances, however challenging. My husband said to me that had I not lost weight, I may not have found the change that indicated I had cancer. He was completely right, and in all honesty, The Harcombe Diet may well have saved my life.' *Helen*

Another Harcombe baby?!
'I was suffering from nosebleeds frequently and migraines that left me unable to see properly. Also I had very painful knees. I could not climb stairs for instance or get up

normally from a chair. I lived on caffeine and high carbs, which I constantly craved. I felt horrid and was about 2 stone overweight. Since starting The Harcombe Diet I have learnt about controlling blood sugar levels and I have lost 2 stone and am now pregnant after a few years of trying! Plus I have learnt an enormous amount about real food eating and found a new lease of life. Thanks Zoë!' *Vick*

I can't recommend The Harcombe Diet enough

'I have done various diets/eating programmes in conjunction with exercise over the last five years, only ever managing to lose a stone or so then putting it all back on in the blink of an eye! I found out about The Harcombe Diet when looking at eating plans to go with my gym routine.

'I decided The Harcombe Diet was quite doable and I started in September 2012 and had an 11lb loss in my first week – this gave me great motivation to continue. I stuck mainly to Phase 1 rules in the first three weeks before moving to a mainly fat-based Phase 2, adding milk and cheese and more recently porridge once/twice a week. After four weeks, I started to introduce my gym programme back in, which consists of CV/aerobics classes two to four times a week and a core strength routine two to four times a week to help with toning. This hasn't really affected my loss in any way. I did have one week when I didn't lose anything, but I put that down to not eating enough as I had been missing meals. I have had some cheat days during the last two months, with alcohol mainly, but try to have these at the weekend as I weigh-in on a Friday. People have started to notice my weight loss, which has helped my motivation even more! I have lost 1 stone 13lb so far and will stop when at a size I am comfortable with.

'Overall I can't recommend The Harcombe Diet enough. I

feel healthier, have loads more energy and find it natural to do!' *Gareth*

After losing 70lb and keeping it off, my GP has never seen me in better health

'I have been gaining weight all my life. At the age of 19 I weighed 133lb and measured 28in around my waist. By the time I reached 46 years of age, I had climbed to 252lb and measured 48in around my waist. Put another way, that's a near doubling of my body weight.

'I won't lie – I ate total junk. Processed food, bread, cakes, crisps and confectionery were my staple foods and my understanding of cooking went as far as turning on the cooker to heat something up.

'Along the way I tried many, many diets, all calorie-restricted and all a complete failure. During each I was constantly hungry, never losing more than a few stone, and they always ended with a rapid return to my starting weight plus a few extra pounds.

By November 2011 I hit 252lb. My overall health was at rock bottom, I was suffering from depression, mood swings, fatigue, tiredness, high blood pressure, acne (at my age!!!), indigestion, acid reflux, constipation, on and on and on. I was in a pretty bad way.

'To make matters worse, I suffered from a prolapsed disc in my lower back. The pain was excruciating and my GP advised that while my weight was not a direct cause, it was certainly a contributing factor.

'This was the last straw for me. I could see that my weight was spiralling out of control and that it would continue unless I took drastic measures. I was desperate. I started researching nutrition looking for something that would work for me and stumbled across the "Everything you thought you knew about food is WRONG" article in the *Daily Mail*.

'Quite simply this was an epiphany moment for me. Whoever this Zoë Harcombe woman was everything she was saying just made perfect sense – finally a diet that I thought I could stick to. I ordered the *Stop Counting Calories & Start Losing Weight* book, read it from cover to cover and started my journey in December 2011.

'Throughout my journey I never felt I was on a slimming diet, never felt hungry, never felt compelled to binge and, perhaps most importantly, saw each and every one of my bad health ailments vanish.

'After three months of the diet, I completed a vascular health check-up, which gave me a clean bill of health, including a return to normal blood pressure and my GP advising that he had never seen me in such good health!

'Nine months later, 5 days of Phase 1 and 270 days of Phase 2, I hit 178lb, a total weight loss of 70lb and unwrapped Zoë's nicest gift – Phase 3!!!

'As I write, I have completed 40 days of Phase 3 and weighed in this morning at 180lb. For me this is the real success story. Not only have I never lost this amount of weight before, I have NEVER maintained my final weight.

'Looking back now the diet seems so damn obvious, sensible and healthy. There are no words that can express my gratitude to Zoë for devising it – she has given me my life back.' *Howie*

REFERENCES

WEB REFERENCES ACCESSED DECEMBER 2012

[1] http://www.mah.se/CAPP/Globalsugar/Risk-Factors/Sugar-Global-Data/Global-Sugar-Consumption/Sugar-Consumption-EURO/

http://www.fabflour.co.uk/content/1/31/facts-about-bread-in-the-uk.html

[2] Ancel Keys, J. T. Anderson, Olaf Mickelsen, Sadye F. Adelson and Flaminio Fidanza, 'Diet and Serum Cholesterol in Man: Lack of Effect of Dietary Cholesterol', *The Journal of Nutrition* (1955).

[3] P.T. Williams and P.D. Wood, 'The effects of changing exercise levels on weight and age-related weight gain', *International Journal of Obesity* (2006).

[4] Dr Kaayla Daniel, *The Whole Soy Story*, published by New Trends Publishing (2009).

[5] W.S. Leslie, C.R. Hankey and M.E.J. Lean, 'Weight gain as an adverse effect of some commonly prescribed drugs: a systematic review', *QJM* (June 2007).

[6] George N. Wade and Janet M. Gray, 'Gonadal effects on food intake and adiposity: A metabolic hypothesis', *Physiology & Behavior* (March 1979).

Finn Molgaard Hansen, Nibal Fahmy and Jens Hoiriis Nielsen, 'The influence of sexual hormones on lipogenesis and lipolysis in rat fat cells', *European Journal of Endocrinology* (1980).

These represent two examples. The evidence is so extensive that the term 'ovariectomy-induced obesity' is widely used.

[7] J.W. Tomlinson and P.M. Stewart, 'The functional consequences of 11beta-hydroxysteroid dehydrogenase expression in adipose tissue', *Hormone and Metabolism Research* (2002).

R.C. Andrews, O. Herlihy, D.E.W. Livingstone, et al, 'Abnormal cortisol metabolism and tissue sensitivity to cortisol in patients with glucose intolerance', *The Journal of Clinical Endocrinology* (2002).

K.L. Morris and M.B. Zemel, '1,25-dihydroxyvitamin D3 modulation of adipocyte glucocorticoid function', *Obesity Research* (2005).

[8] E.S. Epel, B. McEwen, T. Seeman, et al, 'Stress and body shape: stress-induced cortisol secretion is consistently greater among women with central fat', *Psychosomatic Medicine* (2000).

[9] Dr Malcolm Kendrick, *The Great Cholesterol Con*, published by John Blake (2007).

[10] https://apps.who.int/infobase/Indicators.aspx. M. Wadsworth, D. Kuh, M. Richards, R. Hardy, The 1946 National birth cohort (MRC National Survey of Health and Development).

[11] Francis G. Benedict, *Human Vitality and efficiency under prolonged restricted diet* (study 1917, published 1919).

[12] Ancel Keys, *The Biology of Human Starvation* (study 1944-45, report 1950).

[13] Albert Stunkard and Mavis McLaren-Hume, 'The results of treatment for obesity: a review of the literature and report of a series', *Archives of Internal Medicine* (1959).

[14] Barbecue Flavour Pringles.

INDEX

INDEX